Wishing you the
best of
health!

C. A. Foster, MD

STOP
the MEDICINE!

A Medical Doctor's Miraculous Recovery with Natural Healing

BY

CYNTHIA A. FOSTER, M.D.

BREAK ON THROUGH PRESS, LLC
Scottsdale, Arizona – USA

Contact Dr. Cynthia Foster at
PO Box 34693
Los Angeles, CA 90034-0693
drcfoster@earthlink.net
www.DrFostersEssentials.com

ISBN: 1-891173-70-7
First Edition

Cover Art Design by
Toro Design/Jeremy Ortega
558 Waller Street
Unit A
San Francisco, CA 94117
(415) 626-8175 Phone
(415) 701-9653 Fax
jerkait@sirius.com

Printed by
DeHART's Printing Services Corp.
3265 Scott Blvd.
Santa Clara, CA 95054
(408) 982-9118 Phone
(408) 982-9912 Fax
(888) 982-4763
www.deharts.com

Dedication

This book is dedicated to those natural healers who fought to continue their natural practices, despite the harsh criticism, the FDA raids, and other unfair tactics designed to force them out of business. They struggled to defend themselves against the ignorance and greed that kept so many Americans chronically ill over their entire lifetimes.

Those natural healers persevered in their belief that there are no incurable diseases, only incurable people. The patients who had the courage the question conventional beliefs and follow their advice were healed.

This book is dedicated to those who have the courage to look disease squarely in the face and fight it with everything they have – no excuses – *until they win!*

Acknowledgments

I am grateful:

To God, who, in His infinite love and mercy, spared my life so that I could begin to teach others how to save their own. Thanks to all of my beloved patients past and present who may not realize how really loved they truly are.

To Tag and Mary Foster for their unwavering love and understanding through it all.

To Lawrence Minion without whom the idea for this book would still be inside my head.

Especially to Neal Sutz for his countless hours of hard work, editing, and coming from so far away to help me spread the word. Thanks for standing up for me when no one else would. Thanks for making so many sacrifices and for having the guts to take this project on.

To Steve Wolk for his technical expertise and encouraging words, Robyn Weaver for her editing expertise, Dr. Rainbow Casey for inspiring me with her courage, Marilyn McDonald for her understanding, Howard Lyman for having the courage to stand up and tell the truth, Jerry Hart for his amazing sense of humor and encouragement, Robert Matthews who taught me about other viewpoints, Cindy Blessington for her helpful suggestions, Star Townshend for "rescuing" me, Hayward Coleman for etching words of wisdom in my mind, and Joshua Townshend for leading me to the right places at the right times, and always telling me, "That's great!" and to Ron Manwarren for his kindness, generosity and support.

To Michelle Longo for her valuable time, talents, and love, MaryDan for being my most valuable friend in my time of need, and Aaron Elliot who knows how he helped.

To Dr. Bernard Jensen who started this all. Thanks to Michael Pascoe and Brian Carvalho for their countless hours spent educating me, empowering me and facilitating my healing process.

To Leo Munoz who gave me the freedom to be myself under any circumstances.

To Chandni Restaurant in Santa Monica for serving such wonderful vegetarian Indian food with such care and consideration.

Special thanks to Samsonite: major portions of this book were written on a hard-sided Samsonite suitcase since I could not afford a chair. I think it held up very well.

There are so many beautiful people who have helped through all the stages of my healing by inspiring, educating, supporting, and even carrying me if necessary through the difficult times. I could not possibly list them all. My only hope is to give back all the wonderful love and support that has been given to me by inspiring others with this book.

Table of Contents

*Most of the technical and statistical references in this book
come from the Journal of American Medicine (JAMA) and the
New England Journal of Medicine (NEJM), the two most
highly-respected medical journals in this country.*

Preface

This country is finally moving toward the stage of accepting natural healing methods. Visits to alternative medicine practitioners rose 47.3% from 427 million in 1990 to 629 million in 1997. This far exceeds the 386 million visits made to primary care practitioners. In addition, the use of herbal remedies increased by 380%. Patients spent $27 billion out of pocket on alternative medicine in 1997 - a 50% increase from 1990. Despite the popularity of these alternative methods, less than 40% of people tell their physicians about their alternative medicine involvement (Source: Eisenberg, DM, Davis RB, Ettner SL, et al. Trends in alternative medicine use in the United States, 1990-1997: results of a follow-up national survey. JAMA. 1998;280:1569-1575). I believe because doctors are the ones who have the most to lose if their patients use alternative methods, they make it unacceptable for their patients to do anything other than what they recommend. Patients end up suffering with chronic pain and suffering and asking one unanswerable question, "Why am I sick?"

Near the end of 1998, there was an entire issue of the Journal of the American Medical Association devoted to an exploration of alternative healing methods. The question is why is there so much attention on alternative medicine? Why is it that every year, there is more and more money spent on researching these alternative methods? Could it be because they work?! Many medical journals are now including ads for herbal supplements, and antioxidants are being mentioned in research studies for conditions from heart disease to psoriasis. Although a few herbal supplements and antioxidants are a long way away from healing anything serious, the whole world of natural healing will eventually be ripped wide open, and we will all soon discover the truth which has been there all along: that there are no diseases (or lives) that natural healing cannot heal. All we have to do is have the courage to change.

I hope to stir up controversy. I would be very glad and very happy if there were even the slightest changes made in the system. I'll take what I can get. I'd rather have one person healed than no one healed. One life is that precious to me.

In medical school, the professors recommended that we read a book called, <u>House of God</u>. It was an honest look at what the year of internship is like. It had to be sold as fiction, although the author was writing the true story of what happened to him. Some of the stories were so horrible that it was difficult to believe they were real, but they were. If you have any doubts about the difficulties of modern medicine, you might be pick up that book and read it. The author figured out that his patients recovered only if he <u>didn't</u> do any tests or procedures and <u>didn't</u> give them any medications. Since he pretended that he was treating his patients when he really left them alone, his colleagues wondered why his patients always healed so much faster than their own.

This world is so full of quick fixes for health that we've forgotten what a real healing is. A real healing does not just involve a total disappearance of symptoms, but a total change in a person's life - a change so different from the lifestyle previously led to the disease, that the disease could never come back again. Healing happens on so many levels - emotional, physical, spiritual, social, and within the community. I've never seen such healing from a little white pill.

Many people learn when they are healed from a major disease that the disease was the best thing that ever happened to them. They realize why it happened, and what they were supposed to do about it. They searched and asked questions, not only of others, but especially of themselves. They were finally able to summon the courage to do what they wanted to with their life - whether they changed their career to something they always wanted to do, or they left an abusive partner, or they embraced the importance of fulfilling their dreams right now - not tomorrow. I discovered that my disease was an impetus for me to begin my spiritual search. It caused me to journey inward to discover the basic questions of life - why am I here? Why are we all here? Why do people get sick, why do we suffer, and does it really have to be this way? Without my disease, I never would have developed patience, understanding, gratitude, persistence, determination, boundless creativity, energy, confidence, and unconditional love for myself and for others. That must be why my weakness turned out to be my true strength.

I learned many things from my disease. I learned that it doesn't matter what you do. It doesn't matter what you say. It doesn't matter what or who you think you are, you are always loved. You are always perfect. It doesn't matter what profession you are in. It doesn't matter who approves of you. It doesn't matter what other people say. It only matters what you love.

It only matters *that* you love. It only matters that you never stop loving everything and everyone around you. The only question that ever exists is what would love do now?

You can start your life over. You can do what you want to do. You can have a 2nd chance, and a 3rd, and a 4th and a 547th chance. The only one who quits is you, not your chances. Be who you want to be - finally. Dare to take the risk to find out who you are and what you want. Dare to go against the grain of society. Dare to be different. Dare to love it all. And at the end of your life, you will look back, and you'll say, "I've lived life fully, I've done everything I wanted to do; I've had love. I've known joy. I've known tears and sorrow and disappointment, but I tried again, and then I found my true love, my true friends, and my true calling. Then I changed my mind, and did something else, and when I did it, I gave it my all. I did it with everything I had. I faced my greatest fear; I loved my greatest love. I took a blind leap into the vast unknown with full faith that everything would end up all right somehow. I've had a full life and I loved it. So, now I'm ready to go on to the next part." Isn't this the point to it all anyway?

Introduction:

Thousands of Years of Natural Healing

Healing with herbs and foods is not a new concept.

On the other hand, consider that chemical medicines have only been in existence since the 1940's. The concept of poisoning bodies to make symptoms go away has only been in existence for a short while and has continued to grow because of ignorance - ignorance that the disappearance of symptoms means that the health problem has gone away. The symptoms are the warning signals; they are signs that the body is not functioning properly. They are not the disease. Getting rid of the warning signals does not get rid of the disease.

Chemicals are popular because when people have symptoms such as headache, they want the pain to go away right now. Pain killers work well for that and are easy to take; just swallow a couple of pills. When a person has a symptom such as indigestion, they want the discomfort to go away right now. Indigestion? Antacids do a great job of making the discomfort go away; just swallow a couple of pills - convenient for the average American who doesn't have the knowledge to deal with it any other way. Our drugstores are full of chemical remedies that stop most common symptoms - allergies, sinus problems, coughs, colds, flu's, indigestion, insomnia, drowsiness, asthma, constipation, diarrhea, and even pep pills to control our appetite and give us more energy.

Because of the misunderstanding that the disappearance of symptoms means they are healed, people are allowing toxic material to stay in their bodies. When the body is not allowed to cleanse itself through symptoms like coughing, or sweating through a fever, those poisonous waste products remain in the body, leading to another episode of sickness. Eventually, if the healing process is interrupted enough times over the years, so much morbid and rotting material is left in the body that a person will develop a serious disease. It doesn't say on the remedy container that the medicine is made from coal tar and other toxic chemicals. Later, when people have twenty years of toxic buildup in their bodies, they wonder why they have a deadly disease.

I don't have to wonder. I know exactly why. If people only knew how to support and augment their bodies' own natural healing defenses and stop fighting their bodies' attempts to heal, they would find themselves truly healed. They would find that no serious or chronic disease would ever strike them. They would be safe, healthy and happy.

The use of herbs dates back thousands of years. Herbs have been used successfully, safely and effectively for conditions ranging in severity from the common cold to cancer. We find herbs mentioned throughout history in religious books including the Koran, the Book of Mormon, and the Bible. For example, in the Christian Bible, from Ezekiel 47:12: "Fruit trees of all kinds will grow on both banks of the river. Their leaves will not wither, nor will their fruit fail. Every month they will bear, because the water from the sanctuary flows to them. Their fruit will serve for food **and their leaves for healing**."

Genesis 1:29 states: "Then God said , 'I give you every seed-bearing plant on the face of the whole earth and every tree that has fruit with seed in it. They will be yours for food. And to all the beasts of the earth and all the birds of the air and all the creatures that move on the ground-everything that has the breath of life in it-I give every green plant for food.'" It is food that nourishes, strengthens and heals us.

One of the greatest natural healers and herbalists of modern times was John R. Christopher, ND. His herbal remedies were successful for diseases such as anemia, blood poisoning, lack of circulation, heart disease, strokes, cancer, blindness, deafness, diabetes, life-threatening infections such as tetanus, and many more diseases too numerous to mention. Dr. Christopher used to say that there was no such thing as an incurable disease, only incurable people. There are only people who are not willing to take the steps to heal their disease. He has been quoted as saying: "The time is coming (and not far away) when, as our early Church leaders said, the practitioners of medical science will throw up their hands and walk off and say, 'There's nothing more we can do; we are baffled!' And then we'll all go back to the old forms of healing - in the natural manner as the Lord intended."

Dr. Christopher always used to look at the whole body for a healing. He didn't just give a single herb for a particular problem; he was emphatic that the toxic condition of the bowels and other elimination organs were responsible for the particular problem, (the ear infection, the fungal infection, the headache, etc.) Dr. Christopher did not know about the different chemicals in the body - the neurotransmitters like acetylcholine, serotonin, dopamine, norepinephrine, etc., but he did know how to heal any disease with herbs, foods, fasting, exercise, fresh air, water therapies, and other completely natural healing routines.

When I traveled to Germany to learn the water therapies of the famous Father Sebastian Kneipp, I was able to read old manuscripts from the 1800's that were only available in the Kneipp library. In those books, Father Kneipp described exactly how he healed people of smallpox without the least trace of a scar. He described how people would come from all over Europe on their last hope because no doctor had been able to help them. He dealt with severe fractures, cancers, parasites, infections, exhaustion, gangrene, heart failure, and many other serious diseases - all with natural remedies. Father Kneipp took simple bathtubs, watering cans, and garden hoses and effected cures with water of what would seem to most Americans to be of miraculous proportions.

And yet, Father Kneipp was not a doctor; he was a simple priest. He knew how to stimulate the circulation with water, and to use a few herbs, and change the food people put in their mouths to achieve all of his miraculous healings. I'm sure he had no idea what a retrovirus was, and if he did, it wouldn't have mattered to him; the treatment and cure would be the same. Father Kneipp knew that the real healing power lay dormant inside the body, and if the body could be fed properly and supported naturally, the body would go about healing itself. He knew that poisoning a disease out of the body had its price - that of poisoning the body. He knew that a poisoned body can't fight to heal itself. Therefore, no matter what the particular problem was, he used water to stimulate the circulation and call upon the body's own miraculous wisdom and power to heal itself. And heal it always did.

By contrast, modern medicine sees the body as an array of chemicals, hormones, neurotransmitters, etc., governing life. These chemicals govern life. The secret to healing, according this theory, and I emphasize theory, is to force all the chemicals in the body to the right level and there maintain them. If only we could get the insulin levels balanced, the prostaglandins balanced, the growth hormones, the pituitary hormones, the adrenal hormones, the sex hormones, the thyroid hormones, the leukotrienes, the platelet aggregating factors, the clotting factors, the dopamine, serotonin, acetylcholine, interferon, interleukins, stomach acid, and the enzymes, then no one would get sick. Medicine seeks to crutch the body when it's not performing. It will replace what's missing and try to suppress chemicals that are made in excess. The only problem with this theory is WHY ARE THE CHEMICALS OUT OF BALANCE IN THE FIRST PLACE?

Do we have a scientific explanation for love? Do we have a scientific explanation for God? Can we with all of our best scientific teams accurately predict or even control the weather? Can we stop earthquakes from happening? Then how is it that we think we can control the human body? How can be believe that by dissecting it, and giving its many parts different names, can we think that we really have it all figured out?

Maybe it is too daunting - too terrifying to think that after thousands of years of dissecting and analyzing the human body and constructing complicated theories about the body, to admit that we really have no idea why people get sick and why they die when they do.

As I have been exposed now to both methods of treating the body - natural and chemical, and the theories behind each, this book will attempt (I said attempt) to answer that question that has all of the medical professionals stumped. This book will answer the question "How did I get sick and why is it that what my doctor gave me for it didn't work?"

Nothing Stops Love

Nothing could stop this story from coming into being. Nothing stops love - not violence, not fraud, not threats, not lies, not money or the lack of it, not failure, not disease, not contradictory opinions, not cynicism, not indifference, not disbelief and not even lack of faith. Love accepts all of these conditions and keeps on going. Love waits, love is patient, and love keeps on trying until it gets through. It keeps knocking at our door until we let it in. Love waits for its opportunity to love more. It waits for us to recognize that it has no limits. Love **loves** despite our weaknesses, despite our faults, despite our repeated mistakes and our hopeless shortcomings.

I had no idea what love was until I faced my own death. Until this experience I had never felt God, and I had never known health. Natural healing gave me health and it gave me the ability to really love. I knew nothing about natural healing when I entered my first year of medical school, but learned very quickly as the situation in my life demanded it. We change and learn more as we go through this life journey. My philosophy of healing continues to grow as I accumulate knowledge and experience. Sometimes, I want to tell everyone that I know everything. And so many times, I realize that I'm not the real doctor - the real doctor resides within each one of us, its awesome power ready to be harnessed at any moment if we choose to allow it.

As I developed the foundation of my medical knowledge during the first two years of school, the facts I learned about the human body seemed to fit together so perfectly, like the proverbial pieces of a jigsaw puzzle. Everything had a reason or a cause. Anatomic structures are, after all, fairly straightforward. Bacteria, viruses, and fungi infect their hosts. However, as I made my way through the third year of my training, struggling for my own life, while at the same time trying to save the lives of others, frantically gathering, constantly changing data, and working to fit diseases into their nice, neat little slots, I was struck with the realization that there are no slots - there are only people.

People are all different, and they are all affected differently by their afflictions. A patient is not just a constellation of symptoms or a list of differential diagnoses. Each is a living, breathing miracle packaged into a human form - a form that we doctors have so casually dissected and analyzed, in our futile attempts to make order out of the chaos of disease. It's not just disease that's chaotic; life is chaotic.

I was so wrong and so arrogant to think my medical training allowed me to unlock the mysteries of a human body. I was wrong to think that I or any other scientist had the answers as to what **ULTIMATELY** causes diseases and how to heal them. Only our Creator can know these things. So, now as I take care of their bodies, their symptoms, and their pains, most of all I take care to treat each patient with respect and understanding. I accept them no matter what method of healing they choose. I accept their choice, no matter what character flaw I think they have - I have enough of my own. I try to see and expect the very best in them, and to acknowledge that we will all get through the suffering and the discomfort of our ailments by bonding together and serving each other out of love. This is the way it was meant to be.

If my own relatives never take a single herb in their lives and they die one by one from a disease because they don't believe in natural healing, this is OK. I still love them so very much, and who they are is always OK with me.

They help me realize how important my freedom is. I realize how much I want that same freedom for other people - the freedom to have any treatment - natural or otherwise -

without fear of breaking the law, without fear of having their children taken away because they refused some horrible, invasive organ transplant surgery that would've turned their child's life and theirs into a living nightmare. I want all of us to have that most basic and precious freedom - to be able to decide what to do with our own bodies to heal them.

Sometimes, events happen which test our beliefs. I had moved to Los Angeles to practice natural healing and to fight for that freedom. I had crammed most of my possessions into my 8 year-old car in order to make the move, since I didn't have enough money to rent a truck. It wasn't long after I arrived in LA, that my car, however old and beat it was, was wrecked.

I was driving along in the rental car, the one I had been driving since the car accident. I had sold my totaled car for scrap and got a mere $100 for it. They were supposed to save my things for me to pick up, but when I got there, everything was gone - it felt as if I had been robbed. I took a long look at my half-way dismantled car - a dead skeleton. Overwhelmed by my loss, I left, wondering why it was that I was still here, in such a large city where people run red lights and total my car, wierdos try to attack me and I barely made enough money to feed myself, much less make any of the necessary payments on my medical school loans. Not only that, but how would I find the money to heal myself from the serious whiplash from my neck to my tailbone?

I told myself everything would be OK - I knew I could fast, and take herbs and everything else I teach my patients, and it would be OK. But this pain really hurt! Why now? As the tears came again, I wondered, why don't I just give up. I was in a strange city where no one seemed to care if they ran right over you, or if they destroyed the very last thing of value that you own. My 8-year-old car wasn't much, but at least it was paid for. I remember that the purpose for moving here was to get my message out - that people can heal themselves. But, I always knew that if it didn't work out, I had my car, and I could always drive away.

Now, I couldn't drive away. And through tears, I told myself I'd never give up either. Nor would I ever go back to medicine. Not even if I had to sell everything I owned - even if I had to offend people - even if I had to work a 2-bit job where people thought I was nuts. I would never give up my desire to have everyone around me be happy and healed of their diseases. How could I stop that love?

It wasn't easy. I don't like to admit that I had financial aspirations when I entered medical school. I realized I might always be struggling for my last dollar because I chose not to be a doctor who practices drug medicine.

That now totaled car housed my possessions and my patients' files when there was nowhere else to put them. At least I had friends and I had a car. No one asked me why my address was a P.O. Box or why they could only reach me by my voicemail. I didn't have a staff, a receptionist or use billing codes, and all my files were handwritten. Natural healers told me to use waiver forms so that in case there was a dispute, I wouldn't get thrown in jail. I took this risk daily. There was never enough money to advertise, so I worked by word of mouth, sometimes driving for hours to see a patient, if they sounded desperate.

The thing is, all I was doing was teaching people what to eat, what not to eat, how to take herbs, and heal themselves with water, but in the United States, it has not been acceptable to heal serious diseases naturally. Many of my friends and teachers who practice natural healing have been raided by the FDA or even arrested for healing people. It's considered too much of a threat to the medical establishment. It's too much of a multi-million dollar industry for the public to know that they can heal themselves with food, water, and the herbs that grow in their own backyards. It's been postulated that the entire U.S. economy would collapse if we stopped supporting the industries that cause cancer - the tobacco, alcohol, the chemical manufacturing plants, and the medical industry.

I never had a prescription pad or even used an I.V. To help people the way I was doing it was considered

"Practicing medicine without a license" - a license I didn't have and I never wanted. But I preferred that sort of existence over a sterile one in which I injected liquid death into people while I lied to them about the drug's benefits and collected enough money from seeing 50 patients in a day to make myself very comfortable living in a penthouse suite.

People try to be helpful and they think for some reason that if you have a medical license, then you can do what you want. They think a license gives you free reign to practice whatever sort of medicine that you want. They don't realize that a medical license allows you to do only one thing - practice drug medicine exactly the way that you are told to do so. There is no leeway. The licensing boards reprimand and take away licenses from medical doctors who use unconventional methods. I personally know people to whom this has happened, and they were only helping, not harming. So, this thinking that I should get my medical license because I could then have "the best of both worlds" is purely erroneous and wishful thinking.

I've even heard of stories where a natural healer who was getting miraculous results with cancer was forced to move out of the country. There are many cancer clinics using alternative healing methods across the border in Mexico, especially in Tijuana, because they have not been able to practice in the United States without harassment from the government. One natural healer moved across the border into Mexico, and U.S. officials even went across the border and still arrested him and threw him in jail.

This is the risk we take when we attempt to heal people naturally. So, when people suggest that I go ahead and practice murder medicine for another year to get my license, I figure they have no idea how precious life is, how medicine kills it, but how natural healing saved my life and so many others.

It's not a pretty story. At times, it's downright shocking, and sometimes I don't even want to admit the things I found out about medicine are true. But I have to. At first, I didn't want to tell the details of the story that caused me, the medical doctor, to completely turn to alternative medicine. It was much too painful and far too personal. But, as time has passed, I have come to acknowledge the importance of this experience and that it might give hope to so many people who have none. I want people to know that no matter how sick or hopeless or terminal they may be, that there is hope. There is always hope and there is always love and forgiveness. I also want people to know that if they would only try natural healing first, their diseases would not continue to get worse and worse to the point where they're considered terminal.

People do not have to go through the agony of experiencing their hopes being crushed because the medication suppressed the signs and symptoms of a disease only to have that disease return with a vengeance, because the **real** causes were not addressed. What I really hope people to realize is that it is infinitely easier to heal oneself early on before the disease gets to be severe. Early on, when there are mild symptoms, there is not that much to do to heal it; it's infinitely easier than waiting until you've had those minor symptoms for twenty years which eventually turned into a terminal disease. This is the story of how I went up to the very edge of a hopeless and near fatal existence and came back to share the gifts of natural healing. To do this was painful and difficult, as you will read, but it is always possible. Our human will is that strong.

The only reason I have a story to tell is because I and everyone else went to the medical doctors first, got ourselves filled with chemicals and drugs to the point where we were almost dead, and had to reverse all of that drug toxicity along with the sicknesses we began with, with the help of a natural healer. The only reason we waited that long was because we were led to believe that the herbalists and other natural healers were quacks. So, the only reason I have stories to tell about reversing life-threatening diseases with natural healing is because people waited so long to try it. If they would have tried it sooner, I'd have more stories about how cured indigestion, sinus problems, constipation, headaches, and other minor complaints. These are easy complaints to heal with natural healing.

I'm not going to blame anyone for my ill health during medical school except myself. No doctor forced me to eat junk food, to stay in bad relationships, have a poor attitude, or take too many over the counter medications. The doctor never force-fed me baloney and cheese sandwiches, cake and ice cream, and other foods filled with toxic chemicals, cholesterol, saturated fat, pesticides and hormone residues. I made myself sick enough with my diet and lifestyle that I HAD to go to the doctors. The doctors never forced me to live in the big city where I would be exposed to toxic air pollution and other environmental contaminants on a daily basis. Then again, most people never realized that those things were causing diseases - the very **same** diseases that we call incurable.

The doctors **did** diagnose me incorrectly; they **did** give the wrong medication. But, so what? They had no idea what they were doing. The doctors only tried to help. They were merely using the only methods they had been taught, and using the attitudes they subconsciously picked up during their training.

I was the one ultimately responsible for my body and, like many people, made the decision to follow the doctors' advice against my better judgment. I'm not the only one who's done that, and I don't believe that doctors are out there to hurt us, even though I recognize that many medications, procedures, tests, and surgeries do more harm than good. To split hairs, although I accept total responsibility for my health at all times, I cannot accept the blame, either. Psychologists agree that blaming makes someone the victor and the other a victim. It's when we live our lives in a position of having always to blame someone or something for things that go wrong, that we give away our true power. At that point we become victims, helplessly tied to circumstances beyond our control - the actions of other people. The only thing we can control is ourselves, our interpretations, and our reactions to this world. We have to find some way to be at peace with exactly what we've been given, with whatever cards we were dealt in this life.

Nothing is anyone's fault. Maybe we can learn to accept that events sometimes happen for good reason, and that even painful experiences are benefiting us emotionally, physically, and, most of all, spiritually. Perhaps these events sometimes happen for reasons beyond our ability to comprehend. Many people have told me that surviving a life-threatening disease is the best thing that ever happened to them, because afterwards, they learned how to live their life without reservation. They weren't as tied to their fears. They realized the wonderful preciousness of life and that it was to be lived to the fullest. The experience finally liberated them to do just that. I've heard the same thing from people who cared for someone close to them who died. They saw death firsthand, and knew they had better start living. Perhaps a disease is a call to spirit to wake up - to throw off our petty worries and get on with appreciating this very beautiful opportunity we call life.

And death is not failure. It merely is. We are supposed to die, and our relatives are supposed to die. It is that pain of watching our relatives and loved ones die, the fear of death that often motivates us and gives us the courage to go on and accomplish great things. Death is not the enemy that we imagine it to be. It all happens so wonderfully and mysteriously, the workings of life and death, both of them intertwined - the rosebuds blooming, the large oak tree dying, pure rain falling, the eggs hatching, grass growing, sand forming from eroded rocks. How could we be without either? What we can hope for is a peaceful, painless death, and natural healing offers this to us in our last days. When it is our time, we go. There is no negotiating.

I'm reminded of a man who was a patient of my former nutritionist who had pancreatic cancer. He did all the natural healing programs and rid his body of pancreatic cancer. Then, suddenly he died, and the doctors could not determine the cause of death because there was no pancreatic can-

cer left in his body. It was his time to go. Natural healing offers us healing from disease, but not necessarily from death.
Death always comes at exactly the right moment, and new life
springs up out of its remains.

The All-American Dream or Disaster?

Many of us are looking for a "magic bullet," meaning a pill or treatment that requires only a minimum of effort to take, to cure all of our ills. If only it were that easy. We look for the magic answer because we do not understand how it is that we have come to be ill. We think it must be some sort of vitamin, mineral or antioxidant deficiency. Many health product manufacturers have played on our gullibility in this area and have sold us a lot of hype. I have wasted much of my money and time searching for the magic bullet that would cure all my own ills.

Many of us read books, watch videos or listen to audiotapes about how to get healthier. Many of us also intend to make positive changes regarding our food choices, exercise programs, and lifestyle, but later tell ourselves, "I don't have the time," "I don't have the money," "I'm not that sick," or "I'll start tomorrow." Then tomorrow eventually comes, but instead of having implemented these positive changes, we now discover that we have been diagnosed with an incurable condition or disease. We watch as our life-savings go down the drain with all of the medical consultations, lab tests, fancy diagnostic equipment, and surgeries that we think we need. We watch our own bodies deteriorate and our condition worsen as the doctors try the latest and the greatest, new and improved "discoveries" which only prove to be as ineffective as the former ones.

We now discover, to our horror, that our health insurance coverage has been dropped because we are "too much of a risk," and that our doctors want $4,000 up front for the chemotherapy that "supposedly " will save our lives. After placing all of our trust in the assumption that a disease can actually be "cured" by pouring a lot of synthetic chemicals and drugs on top of it, we discover that we have actually allowed ourselves to be poisoned with these substances, that we are suffering from toxic side effects and drug interactions, and that we are actually dying because the medical intervention is too much of a stress on and invasion of our bodies. The doctors may not admit this to you; they merely say that you are dying, but they know better - they know exactly how the drugs are affecting your body.

Synthetic prescription drugs and over the counter medications, which in the short term made a symptom go away or made us feel better, have now contributed to a worsening of our condition to the point where we also have extreme pain that is very difficult to control. Extreme pain then must be managed with more chemicals, and this just becomes a vicious cycle. These drugs have come about in order to make it easier for us to continue our bad health habits - jelly doughnuts, Boston cream pie, steak, candy, smoking cigarettes, taking drugs, and drinking to excess.

I have seen smokers smoke through their laryngostomies (a surgically-created opening in the voicebox) when their larynx was removed due to the cancer they gave themselves by smoking. But, the doctors saved them one more time, so they just kept right on smoking - there is no reason not to if the doctors can keep on cutting out parts and putting new ones in. If the insulin makes the blood sugar level go down, why not eat a lot of sugar because you can? What incentive is there to heal yourself of a disease if the doctor is waiting around the corner to fix any sort of uncomfortable symptoms you have along the way? It is sometimes only near the end of a disease process that the doctor finally throws up his hands and says there is nothing else that can be done. By that time, you may have received hundreds of different medications and procedures that have cumulatively compromised your health.

Most, if not all medications, have side effects. Just look at how big a Physicians' Desk Reference book is - it contains all of the information on current drugs used by doctors. **Most** of them damage the liver and many do damage to the kidneys. Even something as innocent as acetaminophen, which is sold over the counter, has been shown to lead to liver failure. An overdose can literally kill you! Regular use of NSAID's (non-steroidal anti-inflammatory drugs) are also known to lead to kidney failure. NSAID's are also known to elevate liver enzymes counts in persons with hepatitis - a clear marker that shows that these drugs damage the liver. A good general rule of thumb I use is if it has a child-proof cap, then it's too toxic to take. If it's too toxic for a child, it's also too toxic for an adult. If an overdose can kill you, then it's too toxic to take at all.

I don't know of any cases where a person died due to an herbal overdose.

When I was training as a medical doctor, I thought that all of the surgeries, drugs, chemotherapy, radiation, etc. were needed as it was **known** by all of the medical experts that there were no alternatives. My classmates and I liked to think of ourselves as the merciful doctors – almost like saviors, providing comfort and quieting the pain of those terminal patients who suffered so horribly. It was a very satisfying feeling to play the role of the savior. Ironically, though, who would have thought that we as medical doctors had actually contributed to the state of those dying patients, either by neglecting to teach them how to care for their bodies instead of covering up their symptoms, or by directly poisoning them with synthetic substances?

All of the years building up to that cancer, there were various symptoms and maladies, and a doctor could have intervened and changed that patient's life so that he never got cancer. But doctors don't. Doctors don't because even though they know it takes twenty years to grow a cancer, they have no idea what to do in those twenty years to prevent it.

They prescribe the poisonous drugs, and encourage patients to ignore their symptoms by giving drugs that cover them up, and all the while the patient is getting sicker and sicker and closer to cancer and other serious diseases.

When I discovered that there were natural, noninvasive ways to heal diseases and that these methods not only homed in on the cause of the symptoms, but actually improved the overall health of patients, I was ecstatic. I wanted to yell from the tops of buildings that people could be healed, yet I wondered, "Why was there no one out there publicizing these healings?" Eventually, I realized that there were many reasons why this information was being kept secret. I spent countless hours in a nutritionist's office watching those around me heal in spite of the most horrible afflictions - including cancer, multiple sclerosis, Lou Gehrig's disease, severe arthritis, parasitic infestations, heart disease, and many other diseases. I traveled around to the offices of other natural health practitioners to see if they too were obtaining the same results.

What I found was that, in general, people who sought the services of natural healers tended to improve, while those who frequented the offices of medical doctors, in the long term, tended to get worse. Also, the worst naturopaths were, in many cases, actually getting better results than the best medical doctors. There were thousands healed from cancer and other serious diseases naturally. Those who were healed were many times sworn to secrecy. This was to protect the natural healer from getting arrested for practicing medicine without a license. There are so many who have been healed - there are thousands of these people and they have kept their mouths shut. Now, in this environment which is more accepting of alternative healing modalities, many are beginning to open their mouths and tell their stories. This story is mine, but I'm not the only one. And I am not the only doctor to leave medicine because I saw that it didn't work. I am not the first, nor will I be the last. In the coming years, we will hear many, many more stories.

When I realized that it was not necessary to utilize the

horrible, tortuous methods taught in medical school to heal a person, there was no longer any justification for using them. It became an obsolete science to me, and I began to see it as barbaric.

But, this realization did not come without pain. I had to watch my friends continue to believe in what I considered to be cruel methods even though I told them of the miraculous healings I had seen and experienced. I had to watch their disbelief as I became miraculously healed right in front of their eyes and they denied it or considered it a "lucky fluke." I wanted for these miracles not to be true, for everything to continue on as planned, including my medical education. Worse yet, I realized that for me to tell the truth could put me in serious danger, so, I learned to shut my mouth during school hours.

But, knowing the truth involves responsibility. I watched my friends doom themselves to what I considered a hellish life of on-call hours, unintended mistakes they would make that would cost their patients their lives, and the agony of knowing that there was nothing that could be done to help their patients as well as themselves and their loved ones from their medical conditions. I have one former friend in medical school who was told there was nothing she could do about her high cholesterol level because her body just produced too much. I knew that was baloney. Why do we always accept the fact that we have some sort of condition for which nothing can be done? Why do we accept that hopelessness without so much as a second opinion? I knew if she'd follow my recommendations, her cholesterol would be all the way down in 2 months at the maximum and without drugs or other medical intervention. I saw my friends buy into the lies, and because I cared about them, it hurt.

We have been sucked into a make-believe world where "hopeless and incurable" diseases strike us "innocent victims" out of the blue for no reason, and that medical doctors are the only ones who can save us. What we don't realize is that the alternatives (herbology, massage, bodywork, fasting, manipulation, energy healing, etc.) have been used safely for thousands of years and that the knowledge of their efficacy has been deliberately kept from us. We can heal ourselves from and prevent any affliction if we will only take the time and the effort to make changes in our food choices, learn about and take herbs, and practice the same sort of natural healing routines which kept our ancestors strong, healthy, alert, and free of disease. Experiencing my own healing as well as witnessing and being a part of other's healings, I became convinced that as a medical doctor I was harming people and contributing to their early demise.

Upon graduation from medical school, I took an oath to "Do no harm." Because of this, I have since found it impossible to practice orthodox medicine the way that it is being practiced today. I have spent most of my time educating people on the dangers of Western Medicine and on the benefits of natural healing. Most of us don't realize how many rights have been taken away from us and also from our children. Mandatory immunizations are a perfect example. We've been taught to think that if we are sick, it is someone else's responsibility. We forgot that **we actually have the power to heal ourselves**. We've been told for so long that our bodies and their functions are outside of our control that we have actually bought into that lie, meanwhile we vehemently disagree with anyone who tells us otherwise.

We have a God-given right to care for our own bodies in whatever way we choose, with or without medicines, and also, with or without herbs. But, remember we're only issued one of these precious, miraculous, living, breathing bodies in this lifetime. The choice must be an informed one. Will we succumb to man-made laws that say we don't have this God-given right? Must we submit to the invasive surgery or toxic treatments? A friend of mine who healed herself of breast cancer told me that when she refused medical therapy for the breast cancer, her doctor tried to blackmail her. Others have had their children taken away because of a lack of acceptance for natural healing — because not to submit to the toxic treatments was considered, "Endangering the welfare of a child." Will we continue to allow our rights to be infringed upon this way? We will allow the government to take away our children over a difference in treatment options?

When doctors schedule a surgery or other invasive procedure on us, they have us sign what's called an informed consent. This form says that we have consented to the procedure knowing any risks involved and the alternatives to having this procedure done. The doctors never list natural treatments as alternatives to the procedures. But why should they? They have no idea that they work. They have no idea what the natural treatments are - how could they recommend them? There is no natural healing training in medical school. Recently there have been a few electives introduced into many of the medical schools. They are elective, and woefully inadequate. So far, very few students sign up to take these electives. Still, not presenting all the alternative treatments is not fair to the patient. Patients should have the right to know **everything** before they consent to have **anything** done to them.

If the doctors don't tell us the alternatives, it is up to us to research them on our own. No one can really accept total responsibility for you except for yourself. This is such a hard statement for people to accept. It may be the most difficult idea in this book for people to really understand and accept. We are not victims. No one has to help us. No doctor has to help us. We have the ability to help ourselves if we will reach inside and find that strength - find it - I promise it's there! We have choices, and they are always changing, and we are always making more choices that are constantly directing and determining our lives.

Keeping the toxicity of medicine and drugs in mind, let's move on to some of the natural choices out there. Now, we have to understand many so-called natural treatments that don't work. I don't like to turn my nose up at the medical profession only to point my finger at the "natural" industry, but people are dying and I have no choice. Once I made the commitment to write this book, I said it would be comprehensive. I'm unable to hold back my love for people who are sick and want answers. I know what it's like to be hung by a thread, and desperate to find anything - just anything to stop the pain or the disease.

I have to tell the truth.

Few people have the guts to write the truth.

People spend their life-savings to learn about and take supposed miracle "cures," medical and natural that don't work. The results are heart-wrenching. The results of these so-called "cures" usually come to my door begging for answers.

Why don't some natural methods work? First of all, many people misinterpret what "natural" actually means. Natural healing has become a buzzword nowadays. Many things have the label "natural" on them. But just what does this mean? Does this mean that the vitamins sold in the store that are made out of ground up rocks and shells, iron filings, and activated sewage sludge are natural substances that are going to heal our bodies? How do we think that a substance which can kill children in an overdose (synthetic iron tablets) is something healthy for us? Does natural mean the caterpillar fungus, the tuberculosis-filled lung tissue, and spider parts that some homeopathic medicines are made from will heal our bodies? Natural doesn't seem to mean anything anymore. I even see pharmaceutical drugs with the label "natural" on them! Look, I already know what drugs are made from - chemicals from a laboratory mixed with toxic petroleum-based products. Scientists already know that petroleum-based products cause cancer. Some of the same substances are used to produce vitamin, mineral, amino acids, and designer protein supplements. Go to the manufacturers and you will see it firsthand. Many of us who wanted to know the truth have done this.

When a supposed "natural" product doesn't work, this only serves to frustrate people, and make them think that natural healing does not work. But how do "natural" chemicals get us well? There is no such thing as a natural chemical -

it's an oxymoron. Does taking vitamin A made out of toxic, mercury-filled fish liver build new tissue? Do chemicals build new bones and muscles - how about heart or brain tissue? Will they regenerate new tissues like these? I think not! Medical doctors love to get a hold of these fad "natural products" and rip them apart, proving to their patients that they'd be better off in their office than they would be in the health food store. Nothing could be farther from the truth. There are so many natural FOODS in the health food store we could use to heal ourselves, if we would only realize that it takes FOOD to rebuild a body, not synthetic supplements. If we could just fill our bodies full of good food and/or juices every day and live naturally with herbs and other powerful healing routines, we would find that we could rebuild any tissue in our body - no matter what the doctor says about it - no matter if the doctor says there is no "cure" for it.

Let's discuss the word cure. Nothing in this life is perfect or guaranteed. There is no cure for anything. Period. Just because the antibiotics poisoned the germs out of your system does not mean that you are "cured." The use of the word cure demonstrates a complete lack of understanding and disrespect for our bodies. When we put in the antibiotics, we are saying that we have no idea why the germs are there in the first place, that the body has messed up by allowing this to happen, and that it has no way of fixing itself unless given poisonous chemicals. It's like saying that the infection happened because of a lack of antibiotics in our bodies...how ridiculous is that?

Your body is always trying to heal itself. Through the process of infection, the body can rid itself of toxic material that might have killed it. By interfering with this process and "curing" the infection, you have stopped the body from healing itself. Do you really want this kind of "cure?" By "curing" the headache, you have just stopped the signal the body is using to alert you that there is something wrong that needs to be fixed. Pain is only a signal that something is out of balance in the body; pain cannot be "cured" by solely stopping the neurotransmitters from producing it. Why did the neurotransmitter produce it in the first place?

I can't tell you how many people ask me for advice because they're trying to decide what to do about their cancer. They're looking for a "cure." They quote me cure rates for a particular kind of treatment for their particular variation of cancer, and they quote me some kind of number. They might even give me a "5 year cure rate" which merely means the number of people still alive at the end of 5 years - **NOT** a cure, meaning the disappearance of the cancer.

There is no such thing as a cure. There is a life and how you lead it. There are human beings, not our researched ideas about them. If you want to eat junk food, take medicines, never exercise and blame everyone around for how badly you think your life turned out, don't be surprised when you get cancer. But, if you happen to change your diet, take herbs, and heal your cancer naturally, you might consider that a cure. But what happens if you go back to your daily steak-eating, beer-drinking, and other horrible health habits? You're going to get cancer again! Just like how you're going to get cancer again if you get chemotherapy that supposedly "cures" the cancer.

Cancer is not a disease caused by a deficiency of radiation and/or chemotherapy. Poisons cannot cure - they harm. Most children understand the concept that poisons are bad things and they should try to avoid them. We are surprised when it hurts us. There is no "cure" when it's poison. The body "cures" itself when we treat it right, when we give it love and laughter and the proper nutrients.

Everybody wants a simple herb that will heal them, just like everyone wants a simple drug that will heal them. Hey, I understand; I was there; I know what that's like. Well, simplicity lies only in the heart. People can heal themselves of anything if they would only make as much dedicated effort as it took them to get sick and use that effort to reverse that process and get themselves well. You smoked for thirty years? That is a large time investment. You got drunk every weekend for twenty years? That is a long period of time during which you've been hurting yourself. Do you really think it's going to be that easy to reverse all those years?

We still want the simple answer. Why wouldn't we? But the simple answer doesn't do anything for us. It doesn't change us in any way. We don't grow from the experience. Haven't most people tried these gimmick diets that didn't work? What about the easy diet pills? Not only didn't that help, but many of those drugs had serious side effects like irreversibly damaging heart valves.

People pay thousands of dollars to supposed experts, coaches, and trainers who do nothing but talk scientific, complex nonsense to them, teaching them how to fill up their bodies with junk and too much protein and fat. People believe and respect the scientific gobbledy-gook because they don't understand it. They figure somebody very intelligent has already got it figured out. Then people come to me, penniless and filled with cancer, puzzled because they've been doing everything the health experts have told them to do. "I've eaten healthy my whole life - I don't eat red meat," they say. And then I have to tell them the bad news, "But you did eat chicken and fish and turkey and cheese and processed meats, and sugar-filled pastries, ice cream, cakes and pies, and drank lots of beer and wine and soft drinks, didn't you?" Their whole lives they've been swindled for a quick buck by people who didn't have the intelligence or the integrity to tell them the truth.

In one very popular diet book, it says you can eat your ice cream and cheeseburgers, too. Now, what's the author going to say when they come to him riddled with cancer and almost dead from having a heart attack or stroke because they followed his so-called "natural" advice? What's he going to say to the family who's crying over their loved one's bed in the Intensive Care Unit after having a five vessel bypass from following his high cholesterol diet? Is he going to recommend that the cancer patients he created with his high-protein diet take chemotherapy? Then is he going to watch them vomit, lose weight and lose their hair, and say, "but you can still have your protein, fat and cholesterol-filled diet because it's going to put you in that mythical place where athletes perform at their peak? What will he say to the many people who followed his diet and constipated themselves because there is barely any fiber in this so-called eating regimen?

"But I was an athlete," they say, "I exercised every day!" And I find out that they took steroids and ate a high protein diet because their trainer told them they needed all of that protein. And what that excess protein did in their system was to end up as acid waste overloading their kidneys and liver over the years. Now they are screaming in pain with their belly swollen to five times its size because they have pancreatic cancer and they have no idea why. But there ARE reasons why.

"But my bowels work fine - I have a bowel movement every two days - just like clockwork, and the doctor told me that was normal even though I've had these migraine headaches for years, but I guess that's just genetic." Now they're shocked to find out that because their bowels haven't been moving frequently enough for years, that they have colon cancer, and that the toxicity slowly building up in their intestines all of those years was what was causing the migraines. At any point, they could have done some herbal colon cleansing to rid themselves of this problem.

"But my doctor says what I have is incurable so I might as well eat what I want, and besides, my mother tells me I need to eat to keep up my strength." Meanwhile, they're dying because they don't have the courage to go out on their own, do some juice fasting and contradict what everyone else is saying. If you live the way everyone else does, you'll end up exactly the same way they will which is: one out of every two Americans will have heart disease, and one out of every three Americans will get some sort of cancer in their lifetime. I don't like those odds, do you?

Hardly anyone is healthy nowadays. In fact, our entire definition of healthy has changed. For some reason, we think we're healthy if the chemotherapy only makes us vomit 8 times instead of 10, and we can still put in a half day at work We think we're healthy if after the gallbladder removal and the ulcer medication, we still feel OK enough to sit up in the hospital bed and watch TV. We think we're healthy despite the fact that we're on major immune suppressing drugs for the lupus which caused a major infection, but we're still able to make it to our cousin's birthday party. We think we're healthy if it only takes 1 month for the bypass surgery scar to heal - a major surgery involving breaking open the chest bone, putting the body on a bypass machine with our lives hanging delicately in the balance, and cutting the heart with a knife! We think we're healthy if the medical doctor says so, even though the medical tests don't detect anything wrong until years after there were early warning signs that a good natural healer would have been able to pick up on right away.

What the average American considers to be healthy is NOT! When someone with a serious disease tells me that they've been healthy all their life, I don't even begin to believe them. When questioned closely, they recite a long litany of "supposedly benign" surgeries, procedures, and drugs that their doctor told them was necessary, as well as my physical complaints. While they were suffering from toxicity severe enough to require these procedures, the doctor was quick to point out to them that they were "basically healthy." What does a doctor know about "healthy?" I propose that medical doctors know only about disease - they know it very well, but they know nothing about health. This must be why they die on the average of twenty years sooner than the rest of us do. Why do we ask these very unhealthy people advice on how to live long and be healthy?

A Single Hurt Fuels the Drive to Succeed

I had decided to apply to the medical schools in the state where I resided. After grudgingly filling out the seemingly endless flow of forms, writing essays, and requesting transcripts to be sent, I was ready to go on my first interview. This first series of interviews was at a very prominent medical school. I remember how out of place I felt as I kept overhearing very technical medical jargon. But there were some people there that I recognized and knew from college. I remember that lunch consisted of barbecue - not very healthy fare, but it was a tradition there, and who cares about that in a hospital? What does healthy food matter to a doctor - a doctor has drugs in his arsenal to fix any sort of problem.

After the perfunctory tour of the medical complex and listening to all of the wonderful statistics quoted about how many beds the hospital boasted, how many particular types of life-saving machinery and fancy diagnostic tools it possessed, it was time to find the interview room. The professor who was going to interview me, according to my friends, was a great professor who went out of his way to be helpful to medical students and was the type of man who went to the student social functions and socialized with them. What a relief this would be.

As I sat in the chair looking at him behind his desk, there was a long pause while he clumsily shuffled through some papers to find the bundle of paperwork that pertained to me. Suddenly, he blurted out, "I've looked through your application, and I've asked myself over and over, ' Why in the world would this person want to go to medical school?' It just doesn't make sense to me. You have no experience, you haven't worked or volunteered at a medical facility; you don't show me any real interest in the field!'"

I was shocked at his tone because it seemed so cruel. His sexist attitude came out when he asked me why did I not want to become a nurse instead. *I could still help people,* he reminded me. Never mind that I had sacrificed two years of my life after graduation from college to take prerequisite courses needed for medical school that I didn't have because I had not been a pre-med major. Never mind that I had worked full-time and taken classes at night or that I had taken a double course load in the summertime. Never mind that I had to shuffle from school to school trying to pick up those courses that would fit with my work schedule. Never mind that I worked to pay for those courses. I mean, when I decide something, that's the end of it, and I had decided that I really wanted to be a doctor!

Of course, I tried to explain my devotion and my intense interest in the science of medicine and that I wanted to leave my altruistic mark on humanity by taking care of all of its ills. He wouldn't even let me finish - he had already made up his mind about me before I had ever walked into the room. He just kept repeating himself over and over again endlessly belaboring his point. I never requested another interview to replace that one, which I could have done if I thought I'd been treated unfairly. Since at that time I had a tendency to be very critical of myself, I just felt really horrible inside, like there really was something wrong with me for wanting to go to medical school. Truthfully, I was not the typical severely left-brained applicant who memorizes details well and who never questions authority, so maybe he was right for questioning me. I wonder what he'll think of this book.

But then, I grew very indignant. Who did he think he was, anyway? Trying to shove women into nursing, antagonizing anyone with a background consisting of anything except a bunch of science awards and research projects - just who did he think he was? Don't get me wrong, I had plenty of awards and almost perfect grades, but these things did not fill up my life - they were extras. I decided immediately that if this was any representation of what it was going to be like, then there was no way I would go to this school. There were plenty of medical schools in the state where I lived.

A couple of months later, I was accepted to a different medical school four hours away from where I had gone to college. I had decided that this particular school was more friendly. I remember walking down the halls, lost and not knowing where my next interview was, and a few students showed me around and went out of their way to be nice to me. There were many injustices there, too, but I decided to persevere just to prove that first professor wrong. Any obstacle that had the audacity to fall onto my path, I would steadfastly push aside in not-so-fond remembrance of him. It's too bad that he has no idea how he affected me, because if it weren't for him, this book would not exist. That anger was one of the things motivated and sustained me throughout my entire four years of medical school.

Ironically, later on I would begin to heal diseases that the chauvinist professor would not even have been able to touch with modern medical techniques. I'm no longer angry at him; he provided me with a learning experience that I needed in order to sustain myself during an extremely difficult period of my life. For that, I graciously thank him. Maybe he really helped me after all. One day, we will finally be able to see how those events that we had interpreted as horrible or traumatic were really helping us. We just need the courage and the patience to push through to that place of knowing.

The Big Decision -
Leave Medicine or Stay?

At first, alternative medicine was something I tried because I was desperate and there was nothing else left to try. I was hoping that by a fluke, I could get well *naturally* because that was my last hope and I wasn't ready to give up. I wouldn't have cared whether it was natural or chemical as long as it relieved my suffering. So, my only interest in alternative medicine was just to get well enough to finish my medical training so that I could get on with the "real" work of practicing "real" medicine.

However, by the time I finished going through the process of getting healed, I realized something much greater about alternative medicine than I ever could had imagined. I realized that when people utilized the right natural healing methods, they could heal themselves of any and every disease, no matter if they had been termed "incurable" or "hopeless" or even "terminal." I discovered that there are no incurable diseases, only incurable people (people not willing to make the effort to make any changes in their life to get well).

I stand by my decision 100%. Many people ask me why I left medicine. After all, isn't the practice of medicine one of the noblest professions out there? Are not the doctors in our society invaluable, in fact, irreplaceable? They save lives, they manage life and death situations, and they provide comfort and hope to the severely ill. They are always there with a willing ear to provide wise counsel and to give moral support. Modern scientific research supports the efficacy of modern medicine. *But is this really the truth?* During my own medical training, I discovered a different side to being a doctor. Additionally, going through the experience of a life-threatening illness provided me with further insight into how the "System" works.

Not only did I leave Western medicine, but I left a lucrative opportunity to practice alternative medicine because to do so would have meant continuing my involvement with Western Medicine for at least another year. That opportunity involved a nutritionist in town who was the only one finally able to help me after all of the doctors had failed. It was a very sad situation to get well because it forced me to look at the reality of what was going in organized medicine. The nutritionist who helped me also helped thousands of people get well through **only** natural means - herbs, diet, homeopathy, natural supplements, detoxification, etc. But, as I later found out, she was among the many healers persecuted for her tireless efforts. She grew weary of organized medicine trying to force her out of business. She needed some kind of guarantee that her work could continue without the risk of being shut down. I was the M.D. who came out of nowhere.

As her patient, I did all of the programs, and experienced dramatic results. It really was quite miraculous how I was able to recover. Her sincere hope was that I would bring credibility to her work. This is every natural healer's dream. The plan was that I was going to take over her practice. This was a perfect scenario. But in order for me to work with her, she wanted me to get my license to practice medicine. A license would allow me to write prescriptions. Since she needed to taper the medications her patients were taking as they got well, she was dependent on medical doctors to write those prescriptions. In many cases, they were unwilling to do, a refusal which caused many intense moments. The thinking was also that patients might get insurance coverage for the alternative treatments if they were administered by a *licensed* doctor.

Usually, by the time patients come to the natural

healer, they have exhausted every medical method as well as their bank accounts. This, in itself, is a truly awful fact to know that they have spent all of their money and energy on medical treatments that did not work, were misled as to their efficacy, and were even forced to do many of these ineffective treatments. Who stands up for them? Who takes care of them now? I understood her concerns, but I could not continue my training after graduation from medical school. I could not continue to live a lie while putting lives at risk. After having that whole healing experience, I made a steadfast decision never to practice medicine.

Ethically, I was torn. Could one single life harmed during a residency be worth any amount of lives saved in the future by interning and earning more credentials solely to have more freedom to practice only alternative forms of medicine? The whole four year medical school experience had taught me one thing - that no value could be put on a human life - even just one life accidentally extinguished by the increasingly common medical mishaps was one too many. I told her one day that I could never go through the internship - that not only would it be hard on me physically, but that emotionally it would be devastating to do something that I knew would hurt people. One single year. Everyone told me, "It's only a year, and you'll be able to help so many people when you're done." But, I knew every person I would see I could hurt or possibly kill with this system of medicine. My conscience could not bear being responsible for harming even one single human being - NOT ONE SINGLE LIFE.

The worst part is, I knew better - I knew that I couldn't hurt anyone with natural healing - the unspoken miracle healings. During my weekly visits with the nutritionist, I saw and chatted with hundreds of her patients in the waiting room. They told me about how their diabetes was gone, their migraines gone, their arthritis, gone. But the most impressive was the lady who was coughing out a malignant lung tumor. There were the tapeworms and other parasites that were killed and passed and the tumors that came out right through the skin to fall off and be gone forever. I didn't just visit a traditional, run-of -the-mill natural healer, I went to one of the most talented in the country. Rumors had spread of the healings, and people began to come to her from other countries. Seeing these dramatic events on a regular basis made me realize the powerlessness of medicine. I began to view drug medicine as mostly unnecessary.

My colleagues did not share my opinions, but then again, they didn't know about the miracles. The only thing they knew was modern medicine. I can't blame them; they just didn't know. The difference is that *I* knew. *I* would know I was doing harm, whereas my colleagues had no idea there was any way to help people other than the toxic, invasive methods they had been taught. I knew that I would not be allowed to open my mouth to tell my future patients the truth about natural methods they could try, as that would jeopardize the internship. They would surely kick me out of the internship for recommending such "unscientific," and "unproven methods." The trouble is, it's the proven scientific methods that are killing people - even their own research proves that! And as an M.D., practicing natural healing methods would put my license at risk for using "unconventional means in order to diagnose, treat or cure a disease."

Licenses are regulated by licensing boards, and those boards keep track of every licensed physician. By then, I had already heard numerous accounts of how licensed physicians had switched over to natural healing methods, and had their licenses revoked as a result. I learned medical doctors carry even more risk than other practicing naturopaths because the licensing boards keep track of their member physicians, ready to revoke licenses at the slightest perception of using an unapproved method. It is easier for these physicians to lose their licenses than it is for psychiatrists who get caught having sex with their patients. Use of unconventional methods by a licensed medical doctor is considered a *major* wrongdoing.

"Oh, yeah," natural practitioners would say. "Dr. So-and-So used to practice here until they shut him down for practicing unconventional medicine. He was getting amazing results, but, of course, you know that's why they shut him down." It was all very matter-of-fact. Hearing these stories become commonplace for me as I traveled the country talking to natural healers, in search of the truth. I learned because I asked. I asked everyone. This is the only way we can learn. If we don't think to ask, we don't learn the truth, and we certainly don't get answers.

I knew that doing a year of the typical grueling 85-95 hour work weeks of internship might kill me as I had just come out of a life-threatening condition that had plagued me for almost 4 years - almost the entire time spent in training at the medical school. I knew I would not be able to keep up the pace of secretly giving my patients information, as I had done this all through medical school, while constantly living in fear of getting caught. I would make them swear not to tell the doctor in charge what I had just told them, and warned them that the doctor didn't understand natural healing principles, and thus, out of ignorance, would denounce the information as ridiculous.

You see, every time I mentioned to one of my professors the possibility of people getting well through means other than through medicine, it was vehemently denounced as "quackery." Their emphatic denouncing of something that I was seeing work before my very eyes was what caused me to seriously question all of the theories of modern medicine. Something was very wrong with this picture.

Eventually, I learned there was much more to healing than just writing a prescription - I began to discover the emotional and spiritual aspects of healing, as well as the physical, and nowhere in medicine were these aspects being addressed with the seriousness or emphasis that they deserved. Sure I could have done an internship solely to get my "credentials" so that people would listen to me about natural healing and I would be able to collect insurance payments on my so-called credentials. But my decision wasn't based on money. I knew that I could never again be a part of the system and that I would never again be able to write a prescription, even if it was in the name of natural healing.

I did not want to practice halfway between a doctor and a natural healer. *What would be the point of putting a toxic drug into someone, and at the same time, trying to clean it back out with the herbs?* No, if I was going to be natural healer, I would go all the way with that. What most people don't realize is that natural healing, for the most part, needs no complements. People could live their entire lives following the principles of natural healing, and never need to go into the world of modern medicine. For thousands of years, people have lived this way. In fact, worldwide, 80% of the world's population uses only natural healing methods. One could live a peaceful and healthy life that way without ever being scared to death about what terrible therapy is needed in order to control an uncontrollable disease.

I know many people who have lived their lives this way. They have never seen a medical doctor; and if they ever had a health problem, they took care of it either through their own knowledge of natural healing, or they went to a natural healer, faith healer, spiritual healer, shaman, chiropractor, massage therapist, nutritionist, herbalist, acupunturist, reflexologist, iridologist, etc. They didn't question whether or not it would work, they just took care of it and then they were fine. Just last month, someone told me they had healed their cervical cancer years ago with a raw vegetarian diet and an herbal formula. People like that just go on living after that experience, trying to explain to others that - YES - THIS IS REAL! For some reason, people keep thinking a healing is just a fluke, a rare exception to the rule. It is not an exception, it **is** the rule.

I listened to people tell me how I was making such a terrible mistake - that I should do the year of internship, and get a license. That way, I'd be able to do so much more - I could use the "best of both worlds." I couldn't see any good at all in traditional medicine at that time. At the time of my decision, all I could see was the violence, the pleading in pa-

tients' eyes to stop the medical torture, to please stop the horrible tests and the unbearable pain. And, as I loved my patients that much, I could not stand by and do nothing.

I screamed and cried and most of all, I prayed for the
answers to these questions. I had spent the worst four years
of my life learning an entire system of medicine that I came to
realize did not work. Not only did it not work, but in the process of killing an infection or taking out a diseased organ, it
created even more health problems, which somehow people
came to see as acceptable. They just accepted these things as
"normal complications" or "side effects" that never would
have occurred if they had attempted to heal themselves in a
natural way.

I was so angry that no one else could see it but me.
My friends tried to talk me out of my craziness, after all, everyone knows that these diseases are incurable, and if healings
existed, wouldn't everyone know about them, or at least all the
brilliant scientists? Isn't it the job of the brilliant scientists in
this world to know about these things? I was trying to tell
them that they WERE hearing about it RIGHT NOW.
Maybe they thought I was too young and too stupid to know
about what the most brilliant scientists do not; after all, I was
just a doctor-in-training. But, I was enraged by the one phrase
I kept hearing over and over again: "You could help so many
people by doing that year and getting your credentials." They
did not realize that compared to what's possible with natural
healing, medicine was nothing except torture and murder.

If I had gone through with the internships, many of
my patients would have unnatural synthetic chemicals forced
into their bodies in the innocuous-looking form of a pill that
came with a doctor's blessing. Our society deems a pill as OK
as long as it comes with a doctor's recommendation. Every
one of them would experience side effects. Most would experience a temporary disappearance of their symptoms only to
have them return at a later date worse than before, because
the real cause of the problem had never been addressed.
Slowly, over the years, they would require more medicines and

higher doses until they couldn't even keep track of what pills they were taking. They would have to set reminders for them- selves, and carry around special pill cases. Many of them wouldn't even know the names of the medications. Some would even die of fatal allergic drug reactions, either from a drug to which it was known they were allergic, or to a drug that had been given to them for the first time.

Patients would die in the process of getting a diagnosis because the method was too invasive to their bodies. Mainly, patients who died, would die because of ignorance - ignorance of what causes disease and illness. I could not stand it that I would be responsible for these deaths that inevitably and com- monly happen due to the practice of medicine. This is why I considered it murder. I could've taken the same people, taught them about natural ways to care for and heal their bod- ies, and they would likely be alive and well today.

I prayed again. In fact, I remember praying constantly throughout medical school, at first, because of the physical pain, and then because of the emotional torture I felt at having to strike out on my own and speak out against something peo- ple held so near and dear to their hearts - organized medicine.

I wanted to be a doctor because I really wanted to help people. I really did care what happened to them. But I also wanted to be the kind of doctor who didn't have to work so hard - a radiologist. A radiologist, I knew, had the least amount of time they had to be "on-call," and they worked regular daytime hours. I had it all planned out that I was go- ing to have a rewarding career and an easy life. It took a great deal over those four years to pry me away from my perfectly planned life as a radiologist.

The biggest reason I left medicine is because I devel- oped such a love and respect for natural healing and for my patients, that there was no point in doing anything else. Once I realized the incredible power of natural healing and its ability to completely transform people's lives, this piddley playing around with symptoms, trying to suppress them, just didn't appeal to me anymore. Through this experience of facing my own death, I found my attitudes toward my patients completely changed. I am unable to describe how much love and empathy I feel for those who are ill, as I know exactly what that feels like. I cannot deny someone suffering so severely their last hope.

Now I find that I am unable to shut my mouth about how they can heal themselves even though these natural ways are considered by mainstream medicine to be controversial, even heretical. I cannot stand by silent and dumbly afraid of the "Establishment," knowing that if I had only opened my mouth and told the story, thousands, even millions of lives could be saved. We all recognize the power of the written word.

Many people ask me, "Didn't you learn all about disease in medical school?" First of all, yes, I did learn about disease, but I had to learn about human beings on my own time. Also, many people think that once students finish medical training, they know everything there is to know about the human body. Maybe it's because doctors are so careful *not* to let us know when they don't know have all the answers. I did find my training helpful in the sense that I learned anatomy and physiology, and some basic concepts about the physical structure of the human body. I found the experience of seeing patients helpful, as I was able to develop the talent of communicating with people. I learned ways of communicating that allowed people to open up and trust me, so that they would give me the information I needed to help them. I learned about the signs and symptoms of disease and how to recognize and diagnose a health problem. It was enormously helpful to learn how diseases progress when people continue their bad lifestyle and take all sorts of medicines and chemicals into their bodies. I learned some helpful things in psychiatry about how people deny their disease when they're considered terminally ill. I learned the names of diseases and the names of different bacteria, viruses, fungi, protozoa, and parasites. I learned an incredible amount of information in medical school. The only problem is, **all of that information wasn't**

healing anyone. However, it did make me and many others sound very intelligent. Maybe that was the point.

A license does not determine what kind of person I am. A piece of paper does not determine who I am, or what I am all about. I rather like to look at my life as being filled with love for people, for God and for myself. A printed public proclamation that I am acceptable is not required for me to know my identity.

What we are is so much greater than these superficial paper tokens of acceptance that we require of each other. I hope no one blames me for choosing love for my patients over the love for paper acceptance.

The Dark Night –
Is My Life Ending?

This is the beginning of my miracle healing story. The reason I got into this natural healing was because there was a time in my life when I began to realize the tremendous healing power of the body - the power of the body to heal itself, and the incredible, intricate way that the body works. When I discovered this, I was so awed and humbled by what I learned that I decided I had to share my story with other people, to let them know that they actually have that great power to heal themselves. And once I realized this, I began to make another realization that people could even utilize natural methods even to **prevent** the horrible calamities and the epidemics that we are experiencing today in this country.

There are ways that people can take control of their lives and their bodies and take responsibility for the way they're feeling and for the health challenges they're experiencing. By taking responsibility, and doing the programs necessary, they can bring themselves back to health again, as well as preventing diseases from happening.

There are ways to prevent all of the serious killers - heart attacks, strokes, Alzheimer's disease, kidney failure, diabetes, and especially cancer - conditions that are becoming increasingly more common. By following natural healing programs, people can also maintain their current health, and prevent long-term, chronic, slowly progressive and debilitating diseases like senility and Alzheimer's disease, rheumatoid and other types of arthritis, and all of these kinds of diseases said to be incurable.

I knew that there are these ways that people can enjoy optimal health and know that they can maintain this throughout their lives, keeping their alertness and their bodies functioning,their hearing and eyesight intact, and their joints and muscles limber and supple.

By reading this book and learning about the **real** power of natural healing, people will begin to understand that disease is not something created out of nothingness that strikes unsuspecting victims cruelly and randomly. They will realize that disease is something that is being created every day because of the way they are thinking, eating, drinking, living and believing. Hopefully, people will understand that their bodies have the ability, when supported by natural healing techniques, to heal from any calamity, including so-called medical emergencies like appendicitis, poisonous snake bites, many cases of severe physical trauma, etc. I hope they will realize that 99% of ALL surgeries are unnecessary if one only knows about and follows natural healing principles. Yes, this statistic includes the thousands of hysterectomies, tonsillectomies, Cesarean sections, cholecystectomies (gallbladder removal), appendectomies and even coronary bypass surgery.

I didn't always know about herbs, or have this much confidence about the body's ability to heal itself. When I began medical school seven years ago, I had no idea what an herb was. My parents didn't know what herbs were either. We thought American cheese, bologna, sausage and hamburgers were healthy foods. I didn't know the difference between an herb and a blade of grass. I thought herbs were something that were used to spice up a chicken dish. And the only reason I discovered natural healing was because my own health began to fall apart as soon as I began medical school. Healing a body naturally never entered my mind.

As far as I was concerned, every time I or a member of my family got sick, we immediately went to the doctor. There was no way to prevent or to do anything between doctor visits that would guarantee we would remain healthy, or that would give us the satisfaction that we could be doing something to keep ourselves healthy -- other than taking pills.

I just remember growing up in my family, there was always this underlying fear - a fear that some sort of horrible illness could strike one of us down. And of course that usually meant you had to be concerned about insurance companies and whether they would cover this horrible "incurable disease" that you'd come down with. These beliefs were all over the newspapers and on the news every night. We were infected by these irrational beliefs as were all of our neighbors and friends. And then there was always this fear of what the treatment would be, whether that was chemotherapy, radiation, or some sort of surgery. We lived in fear as victims, like so many other typical American families growing up in the age of so many "incurable diseases." We read the newspapers about how such and such person had to have a heart transplant, or kidney transplant. We read the stories about the chemotherapy, radiation, and surgeries and how they made people violently ill.

On top of that, we watched our elderly relatives suffer from these horrible diseases, and later on in my college years, I would watch my grandfather slowly slip away from multiple myeloma, a type of bone cancer. We watched him suffer from the effects of the drugs and chemotherapy. We watched him wither away to a pale skeleton from this disease, when formerly he had been so rotund and seemingly so robust. In a remote hospital in Tennessee, I watched my mother try unsuccessfully to hold back a flood of tears as she watched him helplessly moan from his agonizing pain. Not only did my grandfather have cancer, he also suffered from his environment - his working environment. He suffered from what is commonly called "Black Lung Disease" or called silicosis by his doctors.

All of those years as a coal miner left his lungs diseased and full of coal dust. That left his immune system weak enough to allow a cancer to grow. But the doctors said there was no connection between his lungs and the cancer. In fact, the mining company refused to accept financial responsibility for his death because technically he died of cancer and not from Black Lung Disease. This was because of their lack of understanding of what causes cancer and what causes diseases.

So, we destroy ourselves in the process of destroying our environment, and who pays? The mining company sure didn't. We all pay! The doctors and the medical industry made a lot of money off of it. I know the insurance company made a lot of money off of it. But, I did not know these things at that time. All I saw was sadness and grief over a man lying in a hospital bed with the joy and happiness all drained out of him, who had previously been so full of life.

So we were afraid. Who wouldn't be? What if something serious like that were to happen to you? Do you really think if you deny it and don't think about it that you will keep disease away? Nowadays, a serious disease is COMMON. While growing up, our only assurance that we could stay healthy was that we would go to the doctor when we had an illness, and that we would take our immunizations to protect us from infectious diseases. We felt sure that the doctors knew everything about health, and would tell us so that we could avoid these killer diseases. If a doctor couldn't fix it, we knew it was just a matter of finding the right doctor or the right specialist. Of course, this involved leaving all of that responsibility to our doctor - very easy to do.

And so when I was a child, we really believed in the doctors, and in fact, I went every week to the doctors because I had been diagnosed with severe allergies. I took prescription medication every day of my life and took allergy shots at least once a week from the time I was eight years old. I grew up knowing that someone else always had the responsibility of keeping me healthy, and that person was an expert at doing that. During my weekly doctor visits, I willingly gave my power away to doctors who were considered the experts. There was no reason to heal myself - that was the job of the doctors. I never knew I had the ability to heal myself.

So, I never would have considered myself as the picture of health, but modern medicine had taught me how to **control** all of the seemingly meaningless symptoms - the allergies, the indigestion, the sinus problems, the migraines. My medicine cabinet was crammed full of the latest, strongest suppressors of symptoms that the pharmaceutical companies had to offer. I was always taking a pill for something every day.

When I was seven years old, my mother had taken me to the family doctor because I had been having trouble with allergies. The needles they used to inject allergens underneath the surface of the skin of my back were so painful.

My mother, the nurse and I were seated in a very small cubicle, the front of which was covered by a heavy, blue curtain. The nurse made jokes about each injection - "This one will tell us whether or not you're allergic to hamburgers. This one is for soda pop," she quipped as I felt the sharp sting of the needle going in. In our family, we were taught to be stoic about these things; it was a show of strength not to cry, so I wasn't about to. I remember thinking, I'm not going to be able to take *another* one of those, but yet, somehow I *was* taking them - one by slow, painful one.

All of a sudden, I became very dizzy, and later, vomited. The nurse tried to comfort me, bringing me a clear soft drink to settle my stomach, but the embarrassment I felt, topless and now outside of the private confines of the cubicle, taught me about the harshness of modern medicine. It's easy to make people vomit with a strong enough medical technique that induces enough pain.

When I reached the age of eighteen, I experienced chronic migraines, and chronic tension headaches, so I began to take the migraine medications that the doctors recommended. Also, I developed sinus headaches and sinus infections, and again I took all of the recommended medications: decongestants, antibiotics, steroid sprays squirted up my nose, and even steroid injections.

By the time I hit my early twenties, and started college, I was experiencing a great deal of fatigue. But instead of doing something about this fatigue, I decided to study more hours and even work full-time continuing my education so that I could get into medical school. I figured that whatever was wrong with me, the omnipotent doctors would always be there with their magic potions. Without the potions, I was seriously sick with allergies. Without the medications, I could end up in bed for three days if I spent more than a few hours outside exposed to pollen. In fact, I had a real fear of people opening windows when I was inside because I knew they were letting pollen in from the outside air. When I was in college, my dormitory roommate and I would fight over whether or not to open the window for this very reason. She said we needed fresh air for our health; I knew the fresh air would make me sick.

One year during college, a different roommate and I had our dorm room sprayed because it was infested with ants. I was sick for 4 months with an allergic reaction that kept me miserable, weak, congested, and depressed. I knew the medications were the only thing that made the allergies bearable. I knew the migraine medicine made the occasional migraine pain go away, and I didn't like pain. The allergies could not have existed in my body without colon, liver and kidney toxicity and weakness in my adrenals and immune system. These things a good natural healer could have told me. But they said there was nothing to be done except take their medicines and treatments, and even then, I would still have the allergies, and I would have to "live with them" and "cope." The good news was that the medical doctors told me that I was "basically healthy." Right. Healthy enough to go to medical school. Evidently, taking medications is common and accepted in our culture, and does not mean you are unhealthy.

I've learned that if you need medicines or medical procedures it is **because** you are unhealthy.

And through the years, through all of the needles, the testing, the shots, and the medications, I sought to understand why. I thought that medicine would give me all the magic answers, and that I would not to be a victim of my own

ill health. I wanted to discover the right pill for the right illness that would end all suffering. I wanted to help people out
of their ill health. I wanted to discover the cure for cancer.
Ironic, isn't it - that it's already existed for thousands of years.

And so, when I began medical school and my serious
medical problems arose, I had no idea how to evaluate what
was going on inside my body or what the symptoms meant.
That knowledge belonged within the domain of my doctors.
When the doctors would ask me, in their allotted few minutes,
what was going on and I had no idea. They even asked me if I
was under a lot of stress. Of course, I was so out of touch
with my body, and I had been so stressed out for so long, that
I didn't even realize that this amount of stress was considered
to be excessive. I figured that if I just went in to the doctor
and told him I was sick then the doctor would be able to figure it out. After all this, I figured this was a magical, mysterious complicated process that was far too complex for me.
This process was best left to the ones who were the "highly
trained experts." The doctor would arrive at a diagnosis by
asking me all the right questions and by running all of those
mysterious complex lab tests that I didn't understand. It was
my understanding those tests would tell what was wrong and
they would certainly fix it. Of course, this is not exactly the
way that it happened.

One of my symptoms was a racing heartbeat. I would
have that racing heartbeat. Every morning at 2:30 a.m., I
would suddenly awaken, unable to catch my breath, and a
great sense of impending doom rushing through my body. I
could feel the full force of my heart pounding like a hammer
in my chest. It gradually became more intense each time until
one morning I began to feel that my heart would literally ex-
plode out of my chest. The next thing was a squeezing tight-
ness in the center of my chest that greatly concerned me. It
felt like there was a giant hand grabbing it and crushing it. Because of the pain, I figured that there must be some kind of
damage going on in there. I couldn't be specific - I had just
begun medical school, and we hadn't learned anything yet ex-

cept some basic anatomy. Besides, who expects anything to go wrong at age 24?

We all talk to our friends and relatives first about our medical problems before we go into the doctor's office. I didn't know what this symptom might mean except that it felt like I was dying, so I began to talk to a friend about this, and she told that she had something similar happen to her during the daytime, and the doctor had diagnosed her with something called panic disorder. I thought, in my simplicity, that this must be what it was, so I asked her to give me the name of her doctor so that I could find out. She told me she was taking medication, and that it was helping her. I hoped that it was going to be something easy that it would only involve taking a pill and getting the whole mess over with. I assumed that the only thing I had to do was find the time in my schedule to go to the doctor to get a prescription, and that would be the end of it.

The doctor asked me a few questions, and did a quick perfunctory examination of my heart, taking all of 1 minute. Actually, there were no complicated lab tests to be run this time, let alone any tests on my heart. If he'd have taken more time to feel my pulse, he would have found it to be irregular and he would have heard some abnormal murmurs that I discovered later. I filled out a questionnaire describing these episodes, and I was told that they were very characteristic of panic attacks, and I was diagnosed with panic disorder.

The relief I felt was immense. There was a name for it, and it was treatable. The doctor wrote a prescription for a tricyclic antidepressant, and I began taking the medication. At first, this was a blow to my ego. After all, I was in training to be a medical doctor. Doctors don't get sick- we're the ones who take care of the sick people. And we certainly don't get sick with something mental. However, I was very satisfied with that diagnosis because something much deeper was going on that I was too terrified to deal with.

You see, he hadn't asked and I hadn't volunteered all of the strange things that were happening to me. I suppose I didn't feel them important to mention. I was wanting to hurry up and be done with this problem, so I let the doctor lead me, and since he happened to be a recognized expert on panic disorder, he just so happened to find that I had panic disorder. Three years later, I found the girl who had recommended the doctor in the hall at school, and she told me that she had been misdiagnosed with panic disorder and actually had a heart condition known as mitral valve prolapse.

I just wanted the terrible pain to go away, and I figured that if I did everything the doctor said, that everything was going to be okay again. All my life I always knew that the doctors would make everything OK. I was too terrified that I might have something life-threatening to deal with that fear. Slowly, but surely I found myself increasingly in a debilitated state, and I knew my life was in danger, but I didn't want to admit it.

I hadn't told the doctor about what it was like to be in my body, what it felt like, what was really going on. The reality was that I was barely functioning at all, and that I was frequently on the verge of passing out or collapsing. The fatigue had gotten much worse to the point where I was afraid that if I went to sleep that I wouldn't be able to get back up - literally.

After the nightly attacks, it was becoming a production to get myself out of bed in the morning. The usual alarm clock wouldn't do it anymore, so I eventually had to buy more alarm clocks, to the point that I had 4 alarms going on in the morning, at one and a half hour intervals. I rarely remembered pushing the snooze button, but most of the time I would hear the last alarm because I had set it to the loudest setting of the radio. It blasted me awake, as well as providing such a huge adrenaline rush that I somehow found the strength to sit up in bed.

Eventually, even that method began to fail me, and I had to resort to screaming at myself and slapping my wrists and face. When that failed, I would roll over out of bed onto the floor. I didn't want to get up because my body hurt so badly and because my head hurt the worst of all.

Every movement was an effort, so as I slowly slid to the ground, facing the bed, I used the bed as a support for lifting myself to my knees. With the top half of my body on the bed, I knew I was halfway there. Pushing and straining with arms which seemed to be stronger than my legs, I accomplished a wobbly stand. By this time, I was out of breath, and sometimes I just didn't have enough energy yet to continue standing, and I would fall back on the bed. That felt like failure. *Don't cry; that won't help - I just need to rest a little bit more.* I gave my muscles the commands to move, and they would not. I lay there lifeless with a body that felt like it weighed two tons. I told myself that I had borrowed all of this money to go to medical school, and that **I was not going to quit no matter what!** I hit myself harder and screamed louder at myself. I was angry that my body was not willing to follow my commands. Then, I would start the process all over again.

It became so time-consuming to do this that I would always be running late. When I finally got to the point where I was standing, I would try to run around the apartment in the frantic attempt to get ready on time in order to get to class. As soon as I did this, an overwhelming wave of nausea would hit me, and I would lay back down on the bed again repeating my new mantra, "I refuse to throw up, I refuse to throw up, I refuse to throw up." *Breathe in, breathe out, think about waterfalls, and pink fluffy clouds. OK,* I would tell myself. That usually worked, especially if I took several long, slow deep breaths with it. Because food would make the nausea much worse, I skipped breakfast, except for the occasional glass of juice.

When I got to the bathroom, and began putting on my makeup and doing my hair, I realized that I had to take breaks from lifting my arms, as it greatly exhausted me. As I put on my lipstick, I noticed dried blood inside my mouth. I began to get more and more cuts in my mouth and on my tongue - so much so that soon it became very painful to eat food, and orange juice was definitely out. I kept trying to remember when it was that I could've accidentally bit my lips, the inside of my cheeks or tongue, but could not recall anything. I figured that maybe my teeth all of a sudden had become crooked, and considered seeing a dentist about it.

There was something wrong with my muscular coordination so that every time I picked up keys I would drop them. In fact, I became known among my classmates as somewhat of a klutz because I would literally drop an entire stack of books trying to get them into my locker. I dropped things several times every day. I remember staring at my fingers, trying to move them as they should. It concerned me because I had spent many years learning to play several instruments, which requires a great deal of fingering skills. I think I dropped my keys at least three times every day on the way to my car.

Then began the long half-mile trek into class from the parking lot. It's funny what one remembers. What to one of my classmates was a routine walk into school became my very intense and painful struggle. For my entire life, I had always been a fast walker, whizzing by everyone whom I considered to be "too slow." Call it being a type A personality - I was always on the go, and in a rush to get things done. In fact, I used to think just about everyone was too slow. But then, I realized that I could no longer walk as fast as my friends, and told them to go on ahead of me. While my classmates walked by and passed me, I had a horrible sense that life was passing me by, and that I had become too slow to keep up with medical school.

There was a flight of stairs at the end of this trek leading to the classrooms. I began to dread it, as I could make my legs ascend them. I found the only way to do this was by dragging myself up by the handrails. That endless walk always culminated in an asthma attack. That would usually find me by the water fountain sucking down my asthma inhalers, and later on coughing up phlegm in class. I was trying very hard not to let anyone know that anything was wrong. I was going to be a doctor and doctors don't get sick or have anything seriously wrong with them. And if they did, there would certainly be a miracle drug that had just been discovered that would "cure" it.

Eventually, I was put on three different kinds of asthma inhalers to control the daily asthma attacks. I seemed to be coughing all of the time. The postnasal drip was constant, clearing my throat so distracting to my classmates that they would sometimes lean over and whisper to me, "Stop it!" I couldn't control myself, however, as I was taking the strongest symptom suppressors.

Class was very difficult. It became increasingly difficult to keep track of things. I kept forgetting my friends' names, and couldn't keep track of a simple schedule. I remember asking my friends what class was next, and they would have to tell me three times before I would just give up and sit there in ignorance, too embarrassed to ask again. I was losing my ability to understand simple sentences.

For some reason, though, I seemed to get through class, because most of them consisted of slides, and I could remember what the slides looked like. I had been blessed with a photographic memory and miraculously, that was the one ability I was able to hang on to. My classmates would ask me what I had done over the weekend or the day before, and I was unable to remember anything. I wanted to talk to my friends, but couldn't remember their names, and so I figured out ways to get their attention without calling out their names. I always wondered if they thought me to be rude because I never called them by their names.

I sat through class with my fingers literally holding my eyelids open because I was so exhausted. In fact, I found it a tremendous struggle to hang onto consciousness. It was too much effort. Many times it was too much effort to focus my eyes, and my vision would frequently blur. If I concentrated and put forth a lot of energy, I could put them back in focus again. I had to force myself to concentrate on words that were spoken, and when I spoke, I would forget simple nouns like paper, desk, chair, homework, etc. My friends filled in the words for me.

Maybe they just thought I was too tired from studying to think straight. Eventually, I began to slur words on a regular basis, which I thought maybe was happening because I was trying to talk too fast. I don't know why no one noticed that either. They must have thought that I just didn't get enough sleep the night before. But somehow, I managed to smile and make jokes about it all, so that no one would catch on to the fact that I was terrified and in an extreme amount of pain.

I had slowly developed a severe pain inside my ribcage on the left side. When I had asked the doctors about it, and the answer had been "I don't know what that pain is." Again, they told me they thought I was basically healthy. If I turned in a particular direction, I could actually feel something swollen in there scraping up against my ribcage. I persevered through class, eventually taking some sort of painkiller every day. I wondered if it could be harmful to my kidneys and liver to be taking so many painkillers. The constant pain made it very difficult to breathe, but I told myself that since no doctor thought anything of it, everything was okay. After all, I was *basically healthy*. Since everything was okay, that meant I could just continue this way and probably the pain would just go away. I've always marveled at how strong denial can be in other people, and I've just recently come to appreciate the strength of my own during that trying time.

But, the pain **didn't** go away. Because of that pain, and the chest pain, and the neck pain, I was always holding my ribcage, my chest, or my neck, and I suppose I was very good at making it look like either a nervous gesture or a sexy pose, so no one suspected the amount of pain I was experiencing. The pain in my legs was constant which felt somewhat like the flu, and I began to wonder if maybe I had some sort of chronic viral infection like Chronic Fatigue Syndrome. I figured the neck pain was some sort of chronically swollen lymph nodes, and since I knew people with Chronic Fatigue Syndrome had this problem, I figured I must have CFS. However, there were no swollen lymph nodes on the left side of my neck, only the referred pain from the heart problem.

Midmorning, the hot flashes would come and I'd break out into a sweat. My friends would tell me I looked pale, and I'd feel weak with hunger. I figured out how to deal with this was to go to the vending machine and get a candy bar. I ate so much sugar to keep up with this that it was a topic of conversation among my friends. One of them even offered to get me bulk size of chocolate candies at the food warehouse, which I accepted. I could not get enough food to satisfy my hunger. I began to eat large amounts of food. My friends were jealous because instead of gaining weight, I was losing it. One time, the vending machine ate my nickel when I had gone to the machine with only the exact change. I started crying and going nuts over the fact that I couldn't get something to eat because I was "starving." Some nice man gave me a nickel, and I became sane again after I had my sugar fix. Who says sugar is not a drug?

Thank God, the first two years of school were lectures. All I had to do was sit for those. . No one seemed to notice how unsteady I was on my feet. I just had to make sure when I stood up that I had something to lean on. This really wasn't too difficult to hide from people.

Walking back to the car after class was easier, as it was all downhill, but that would usually be the last time during the day that I could walk. I came in the door of my apartment and collapsed on the floor. Around three hours later, I would wake up, startled by the sound of the phone. I would crawl to the phone, the effort leaving me out of breath, and answer it.

It was Edward. Thank God, Edward called me so often, otherwise I truly might not have woken up until the next day. Actually, the real reason Edward called me so often was because he liked me. He wouldn't admit to it, as he was living with his girlfriend at the time. But, all I know is that he kept calling and wanting to spend time together, and he was also telling me about all of the problems he was having with his girlfriend at the time. Regardless of the reason, it was a very good thing for me that he did call so often. It kept me conscious at least part of the time.

When he called, he always asked me why I was so out of breath, and did I just run to get the phone? He didn't know that just the act of crawling put me out of breath. I always just said yes. I had no idea why I was so out of breath; it was easier to just let it slide. For some reason, he never caught on. He knew that every time he called me, he woke me up, but I guess he figured that I had stayed up all night studying, and that it was normal for me to have an afternoon nap every day. It's not too uncommon for medical students to "pull an all-nighter". I don't think he knew my daily nap lasted *over three hours*, though.

After the phone rang, I realized that a lot of time had gone by, and that I had no idea what had happened. I some-times would say things to Edward on the phone and later for-get what I had said, causing many misunderstandings between us. I had to ask people frequently to repeat themselves, so that I could understand what they had said. Once, we were out to dinner in a group, and Edward and his friends were discussing something that I simply could not follow. When asked to pro-vide my opinion about it, I couldn't because I had no idea what they had been talking about. I was trying to listen, but it just took too much effort for me to understand the words. He accused me of not listening on purpose. In fact, he was able to explain my memory lapses and inattention away as being be-cause I was acting "ditzy" and just trying to be accepted.

His intended specialty as a student was psychiatry, which explains all his "theories" about me. Since intelligent people can have a difficult time being accepted socially if oth-ers think of them as brainy nerds, and hate it that they do well on tests, he thought I was acting ditzy on purpose, in the hopes of being more popular. At that point, winning a popu-larity contest was the least of my concerns. Sometimes, he even made jokes about how I acted in such a ditzy manner. Since he knew I had been diagnosed with this mental disorder, he probably was able to explain away my so-called physical symptoms as being "all in my head." He did not do it on pur-pose - he was just acting according to what he had been taught in medical school.

     Organized medicine teaches us to think that disease is only mental or only physical and never anything in between . It's this mind-body split in Western Medicine that has caused so many people so much suffering. Once you're diagnosed with something mental, you can just forget about any doctor or doctor-in-training to ever take you seriously about any physical symptom you have. Your physical state is going to be pretty much ignored and symptoms you have will be explained away as not being real because you made them up because you're "hysterical." On the other hand, people with serious so-called physical diseases are led to believe that there are no emotional issues to deal with, so they don't deal with them, and consequently, miss a large contributing factor that caused their "physical" disease. Both doctors and patients miss a tremendous healing opportunity.

     Some days in medical school were not so bad, but I would also have lucid moments. I would occasionally spend time with friends, go to parties in the evening or even go out to dance during the first several months of school. One night I was at a popular nightclub and medical school hangout celebrating the end of a series of tests. I was feeling pretty tired, but otherwise fine, until I had two margaritas. All of a sudden, the left side of my neck hurt so intensely I couldn't help but to hold it. I was almost crying. I asked my friends what they thought it could be, and of course, they didn't know, either. Eventually, I figured out that drinking alcohol made the pain worse, so I stopped drinking. It wasn't hard once I understood the connection. Alcohol harms the body and harms a sick body even more. Forget our wishful thinking about the healthy benefits of drinking red wine, this was real life, not some ill-conceived research study. It was aggravating my heart, sending the pain up my neck.

     Most of the time, I made up excuses to my friends about why I couldn't go out. "I have to study" was my favorite. All the medical students could relate to that one. Sometimes people would notice that I wasn't feeling well, and ask,

"Are you feeling okay?" My usual response was, "I'm fine; I'm just tired, that's all." Everyone believed me. Maybe they thought I was studying constantly and was never taking a break, and that's why I seemed so tired and out of it. Although I was sleeping up to 14 hours a day, when I was awake, the only thing I would do was study and eat. I found this the only way to get decent grades, considering I lost so much time every day being unconscious from the seizures that I didn't know I was having at the time.

During those months, I tried to get healthier, thinking that it would help me. I had lost some weight, and I figured if I could just put it back on that everything would be okay again. Trying for that simple answer again. Now I know that putting on weight has nothing to do with being healthy. But back then, I went to the store and got the athlete's drink mix in a powder that had the most calories (2,000 to be exact). I hated that stuff. It always nauseated me. I finally grew tired of the protein shake that did nothing to heal me or help me gain weight.

The apartment complex where I lived had a large workout facility, and I figured this would be a great way to gain weight. I had always been athletic except for the past few years, so I thought it would be a piece of cake. For some reason, though, my body did not see it that way. Near the end of my workout, I would begin to black out. I could see the black rapidly closing in, and I knew I was going to collapse, and I would immediately stop what I was lifting. That really scared me. Luckily, I never fell. I was too afraid after a few of these incidents to go back to the gym. It was too frustrating. I didn't know it was because of my heart.

Meanwhile, the migraines came more frequently and more intensely. I asked one of my friends to get me a prescription for codeine (a powerful narcotic pain reliever) so that I could handle the pain of the migraines. It would be hard to describe the pain of the migraines in words, but they made me go out of my mind. I would bang my head on the floor and against the wall to distract myself from the pain. I would scream into my pillow with every last bit of energy in me until I completely exhausted myself. I screamed at God for cursing me with this unbearable pain and why had he put me on this world to suffer this way? After all, I was not a happy sick person, so I fought it every step of the way. I was angry that he had left me alone and abandoned. I repeated the prayer, "Please God make it stop, make it stop, make it stop....Why won't you help me? You know I can't take any more of this pain!"

When I was exhausted with that, I would try to bargain with God to make the pain stop - I would promise all sorts of things. But, that never worked either and I would cry very weakly. But, crying, I found out, made the pain worse. Then I begged God to please take my life and let me die. I didn't know how it was possible to still be alive and have that much pain at the same time. I figured that much pain would probably kill a person, and I wondered why I was not dead already. I had no idea what was going on around me; all I could think about was the pain - every single minute - the pain, more pain, and more pain. Can I make it another minute with this pain? Over and over I would plead, God, please help me make it for one more minute. Maybe God was too busy to help me deal with this pain, so I prayed to every Catholic saint I could think of. I prayed to the Virgin Mary, I prayed to the Holy Spirit, and I prayed that God would send me a guardian angel to protect me and help me with the pain at all times. I figured the job was too big for just one guardian angel, so I asked for two. That way, they could switch shifts when they got tired. Sometimes, the thought that I was being protected was the only thing that kept me going.

Although many times I was suicidal, something inside me wanted to survive. Part of me wasn't finished with this life - I thought I was just too young to die, and I had never done anything important in this life. A person's life just can't end this early, I thought. A person who's 24 has barely begun life. I never had a career or a family. I hadn't traveled that much - I hadn't truly seen the world. I grieved at the thought of losing my life, and losing the experiences that I thought I'd never have. This disability was affecting my life negatively, and it upset me unnecessarily.

As I couldn't walk much, I devised a way to go about life in my apartment by crawling. All of the medical books I kept on the floor. I would frequently wake up in the middle of the nights with my hand still clutched around my highlighter, having used every bit of energy I had just to understand the last paragraph I read. Eventually, I learned how to use counters and handles to pull myself up to standing. When I was too tired to crawl, I would roll - that was easier.

In fact, I was so weak, that even chewing became an effort, and I began to choke during my meals. I discovered that I needed to take rest breaks from chewing.

"I used to be able to do this!" I would scream inside my head as I would read a paragraph over and over and could not comprehend the words. It didn't seem to matter what the subject matter was, I had to work harder than I ever had at everything I did. I could feel my brain function slowly slipping away, more and more with the passing of each hour. I felt that I must be going insane. When I heard people speak, I knew that it was words coming from their mouths, just not what those words all meant together as a sentence. This was particularly devastating as my mind was something I had previously always been able to count.

Because my hands would not move in a coordinated way, I fought to make the buttons go through the buttonholes of my shirts. *I don't have time for this. I'm going to be late. I'm losing all my abilities. I'm losing everything!* I prayed and prayed, struggling with the thought that a serious hidden disease was slowly sucking away my life, and it was.

I was increasingly losing my ability to do even the small things like comb my hair, change into my pajamas, brush my teeth, do the laundry and dishes. Even standing in the shower was becoming too much of an effort.

My parents lived out of state, and although I was in touch with them occasionally, nothing ever came up except

that I stated that I didn't feel well. Bless my mother's selfless-
ness. She told me that if I ever needed to, I could always
move back home with her. It's not that I didn't love her, but
to have given up school would have been like failure. I didn't
want to disappoint my parents. In fact, the whole family was
so proud of me, that my two brothers started to express interest in becoming medical doctors, as well. I felt like everything
hinged on me to be the one in the family to "make it" by becoming the successful doctor.

The Last Straw

So, I continued to go to different doctors hoping that someone would find what was really wrong, but to no avail. Once a diagnosis of a mental disorder (panic disorder) is written in your medical chart, no one takes you seriously anymore. The doctors would look at my chart, look at me, pat me on the head, and tell me there was nothing wrong. I never had any real lab tests or a thorough history or physical taken, just a funny smile like I was just hysterical or maybe even making things up.

Quite ironically, someone had found the problem with my thyroid during my second year of school. We were learning how to do physical exams in small groups. As I was the guinea pig of the week, the instructor was showing how to palpate the thyroid on me. When she touched it, I screamed. It was very painful. She looked me in the eye and said, "You'd better have your thyroid checked." But she was too late. The doctors I had seen had all convinced me that I had this anxiety disorder, and I had heard it so many times that I believed it. Besides, I didn't want anything wrong with me; I would rather have had a simple anxiety disorder - even as stigmatizing as it is to have a mental disorder.

One doctor told me the problem was that I had globus hystericus, which is a glorified medical term for feeling a "lump in the throat." Hystericus is the Latin word - guess what it means - that this feeling was all in my head. I really had a swollen thyroid due to severe Grave's disease. Another doctor told me I had irritable bowel syndrome (again because of the thyroid problem). Another told me I had a sleep disorder and an anxiety disorder. Another told me I might have cancer of the lymph nodes. It turned out not to be that, and I narrowly escaped a lymph node biopsy.

One doctor actually screamed at me because I told him I was waiting to be approved for medical insurance, and he practically booted me out of his office. He never even asked me, but at that time, I could've paid out-of-pocket anyway. He wasn't interested in listening. He was too busy on the phone discussing the details of his new, very expensive car. This same doctor insisted on ordering a pregnancy test, even though I told him that there was 0% chance of this, considering I was celibate at the time. The reply is still etched in my mind: "A good doctor never takes the patient's word for it; he always has to assume they could be lying." That was so demeaning.

I walked out of his office and into the parking lot, unable to hold back the avalanche of emotion from having been yelled at like a naughty child. His abrupt, intimidating manner cut right through me, and I burst into tears. Every time I tried to get a diagnosis, I received a wrong one and then was humiliated on top of that. Ironically, that same day, the approval for my medical insurance came in the mail, meaning I would have been covered for the visit anyway.

The doubts came up - would I live or die? I was so terrified I couldn't handle it anymore. I prayed again - Will I never be well again? And lying there on the floor in front of the door of my apartment where I had collapsed after coming home from school, I lost consciousness on top of my Bible. God was the only thing I could hang onto. It was the middle of the afternoon. In the wee hours of the night when I awoke, I heard it as clear as a bell, "Your weakness is your strength."

I lifted my chin off of the Bible and thanked God for what made no sense to me at the time. Utterly exhausted and unable to budge from the spot, I went back to sleep and stayed there all night. How was I losing so much time out of the day? I would have to try harder tomorrow to stay awake.

It was not something I wanted to do - see a psychiatrist, but my doctor told me that I needed to go because of the supposed panic disorder. I was able to appear mostly normal in front of the psychiatrist. All I had to do was sit - I didn't have to stand to do anything; sitting was so much easier. All I had to do was get to my car and back, and the rest was just sitting and trying to speak, paying attention and keeping my eyes in focus.

It wasn't so bad actually - I complained about all the love I didn't get as a child, and I delved into my inner child. I could see he didn't believe me when I told him I couldn't remember much about my childhood. Of course he had no idea I had a hard enough time remembering what I had done two hours ago. Still, I felt somewhat less anxiety about things, and I had something to go to once a week that was stable, which was important to me since everything else in my life was reeling out of control. So, I began to feel more at peace about my childhood and able to forgive my parents for what I thought they should or shouldn't have done. I remember telling him that I thought I was feeling much better. But I really was just wanting so badly for it to be true that I was just deluding myself.

Physically, I was still a wreck, but the psychiatrist just took my doctor's word for it that I had this mental disorder. I remember telling him that I was having a difficult time walking up stairs. He seemed to think it was because I was merely depressed. At that point, he wanted to increase the dosage of my medication. But something inside me screamed NO! That was the second time I got some sort of inner wisdom, and I wasn't going to ignore it.

Since I had begun the medication, life had gotten even more bizarre. I began to spontaneously hear music that I had played years before in concert band. I could hear the music note by note - every minute detail, every nuance, every crescendo and decrescendo. I began to hear peoples' voices in my head from conversations I overheard during the day. They weren't telling me to do anything, but the constant internal chatter made it very difficult to listen to people on the outside. I would wake up in the middle of the night, but instead of the chest pain, I would outright hallucinate. I would misinterpret the shape of my closet, and it became something very scary to me. A hook on the ceiling turned into a moving spider. At times, I would wake up and I would literally be paralyzed - I could not move a single muscle. I eventually got to the point where I was so terrified of these episodes that I could no longer go anywhere near my bed, much less sleep in it. I began to camp out on the couch with my pillow and blanket. For a while, this seemed to lessen the frequency of the attacks, so my simplistic mind figured that there must be something wrong with my bed.

The episodes continued full force, at which point I developed a phobia of sleeping. All day long I would fight to stay awake against the exhaustion, and all night long I would fight to keep awake because of the fear of going to sleep. I knew that whenever I went to sleep, bad things would happen. I finally reached that point where something inside me screamed, "This is too severe to be panic disorder; this is something else!"

There was a day when the chest pains were particularly bad. My heart was jumping around throughout all of my classes, and I felt a very uncomfortable sensation in the center of my chest. After an argument I had with one of my lab partners about something completely trivial, she wanted to vent a lot of anger. I was upset, and left the room. As soon as I did, however, the crushing pain came down on my chest. It was as though all of the air had been forcefully expelled from my lungs with a vise, and no air could get back in. I gasped, but was unable to speak during these minutes except for a slight whisper, "Ow...ow...ow...ow..." The pain almost dropped me to my knees. Just outside the door, I stood alone taking in only empty gulps of air, gasping and clutching at my chest.

One of my classmates came out and she asked me what was happening. As I was still trying to hold it all together, I told her it was nothing to worry about. She was very worried and told me that I needed to see a doctor immediately. In as calm a tone as I could muster, I told her that I had already seen the doctor, and that he seemed pretty convinced that it was this "panic disorder" diagnosis. She didn't seem as convinced as the doctor, and if the pain had not gone away in a few minutes, I think she would have called an ambulance. At that point, the ambulance would've been good for me. The doctors would've found something wrong. But I did not want to make a fuss. It was just like me to deny the obvious - that I was seriously ill and could not go on much longer this way.

One morning I woke up with my shoulder out of its socket. It was an unbelievable pain. Panic-stricken, I rushed to try to push it back in to relieve the pain as soon as possible. There was absolutely no doubt that it was out; the sensation was unmistakable. I realized that I was going to have to push harder and to try pushing in all different directions. Through trial and error, I pushed with all my might, frantically trying to get it back in because of the intense discomfort. Finally, I heard a crunch, and the sensation of my shoulder going back into the socket. The pain was immediately relieved.

I didn't know why this had happened, so I went to the doctor. The doctor looked at my chart, with that mental diagnosis already in it, and looked at me. He told me I had probably just heard the sound of my tendon brushing up against my bone, and that I should take some aspirin, then put a warm compress on it. I think I was so relieved to know that I had not done any permanent damage to my shoulder, that I expressed nothing but thanks in response. Truly, he just confirmed what I really wanted to hear - that there was nothing seriously wrong - I was basically healthy! Not wanting to consider myself a wimp, I took neither aspirin, nor a warm compress.

The dislocations continued, and I began to become expert at the particular angle and force needed to push it back in. I told myself that this must be happening because I slept on my stomach.

Many doctors would consider it malpractice not to investigate the cause of something like that. Dislocating a shoulder during sleep does not happen to people who are well. It is a sign of something very serious. However, that doctor did not seem to be concerned at all about finding out what caused my shoulder to be dislocated.

What was really going on was that I was having the most severe sort of epileptic seizures - called grand mal seizures. The force of the muscular contractions during these seizures are powerful enough to dislocate joints and even fracture bones, but seizures were something my doctor never considered because he figured I made the whole story up, since I had been previously diagnosed with an anxiety disorder.

A person who has this type of seizure very commonly injures himself during the seizure - whether it's a pulled or strained muscle, a dislocation, bruises or cuts in the mouth as a result of the jaw muscles going into spasm and the teeth grinding down full force on the tongue and the insides of the cheeks and lips. People have even been known to bite off the tip of their tongue during an epileptic seizure. Luckily that never happened to me.

Some epileptics get early warning signs that a seizure is about to happen. These are called prodromal symptoms, or an "aura." An aura can be anything like a feeling of a rising sensation in the gut to hallucinations - hearing and seeing things that are not really there.

So, I never knew what to expect when I woke up. Several times I would wake up in tremendous pain as I caught the tail end of a seizure. I would check my mouth for cuts, and move everything around to see if I had pulled or dislocated something. That became my morning ritual. I didn't know what seizures were back then, so I still had no idea that I was having them, just that these things happened to me every time I went to sleep. The doctors suspected nothing. Seizures didn't run in my family, and I didn't know anyone who had them. Later on in my training, though, I would actually see patients with seizures, interview them, and make recommendations regarding their medications, etc.

A person can have seizures without being aware of them, so no one knew that I was having these, least of all me, because they always happened when I was sleeping or unconscious. Since I lived alone, no one ever saw me having any seizures. Later I realized that I was also having the petit mal seizures throughout the day, where I would just space out for several seconds and miss what was going on.

After a grand mal seizure is over, people are exhausted. Their muscles hurt, they have a headache and nausea, and all they want to do is sleep. Immediately after the seizure, a period of confusion follows which lasts anywhere from a few minutes to a few hours. Fine motor coordination (finger dexterity) is also affected for a short period of time after a seizure. During a grand mal seizure, the entire brain just shorts out, due to a surge of electrical activity that causes the seizure. I remember sometimes it would feel like my brain had been electrocuted, like I had stuck my finger in an electrical socket, and the shock went to my brain. The surge of electrical activity causes the body to go into a hyperactive state - the characteristic rhythmic spasms that we observe in epileptics.

Because the brain shorts out, it cannot function properly, and memory is affected. Many times I would be sitting in front of the psychiatrist and I would lose my ability to understand what he was saying. I would just stare into space. When asked about this, I would tell him, "My brain is too tired to think," but I don't think he believed me. The truth was that my brain was so fried from having so many seizures that many times I would have no thoughts at all. He told me, "People don't just think about nothing." Maybe he figured that I must have been thinking about something and just hiding it from him.

Actually, it wasn't so bad having periods of no thoughts at all. There was absolutely no stress to it. My thoughts were slowed down so much, it was almost as if I spent a large part of the day in a deep trance. It's very good that that happened, otherwise I would not have been able to handle the intense pain and disability I was facing every day.

You could call it God's special blessing to me that I inadvertently cursed him for.

My excuse for all of this was that it was just the stress of medical school and I had used the "mental disorder" diagnosis to explain away the alarming symptoms, insisting to myself that the doctors must be right, and that they knew exactly what they were doing. I even cracked jokes about being diagnosed with "this mental thing." It was much easier to let someone else take the responsibility for my condition - the doctors are taking care of it with this medication. Responsibility for myself was something I would soon learn.

Since the doctors didn't know I was having seizures instead of panic attacks, they put me on that antidepressant instead of anticonvulsants (medicines used to treat seizures). Unfortunately, synthetic drugs do not come without their side effects. This particular kind of antidepressant had side effects: one that affected heart rhythm and that lowered the seizure threshold, thereby making it more likely to have a seizure. Since I was already having them, it had stimulated in me even more seizure activity, causing all of the very bizarre symptoms.

It's no surprise to me now that the medication had stimulated more seizure activity, but at the time, I fully trusted the doctors to give me the right medicine to heal me. I never suspected the doctors could actually have made my condition much worse. But, I was the one who let them and I take responsibility for that.

My doctor had not been completely truthful with me about the side effects of that medicine. I had told him I had a very important physiology test coming up and asked if the medicine would help me to feel better. What he didn't tell me is that in many cases, symptoms are aggravated even more as the body adjusts to the medication. It just would have been nice to know that. What happened is that I walked into the physiology test feeling more chest pain and more terror that ever before, completely unable to think or concentrate, and consequently missed failing the test by one point. I went home and while lying down on the floor, doing absolutely nothing, felt my pulse speeding at 140 beats per minute. It stayed that way continuously for one week while I "adjusted to the medication".

It also worsened my blood pressure to the point where every time I stood up, I almost passed out. No one told me that those tricyclic antidepressants are known for causing liver function test abnormalities, meaning that they damage the liver. Damage to my liver, I would later find out when learning about natural healing, was actually perpetuating and worsening the problem. It was allowing me to stay sick and get worse. I guess no doctor ever felt it necessary to mention that tricyclic antidepressants can actually cause psychosis - hallucinations, etc. The drug constipated me (as do all tricyclics and many other drugs) which helped my body to retain more and more poisons that would contribute to a worsening of my condition.

Something inside finally screamed NO!

I knew that the really bizarre events coincided with the time I first began the medication.

Meanwhile, the student clinic family doctor who had first diagnosed the panic disorder decided to change me to a different medication. It was one that was being introduced as a new treatment for panic disorder. He did that because I told him that the chest pain was not going away. Instead of the short, intense episodes, I was now having a dull, almost constant pain in the center of my chest with not as many intense episodes as before on top of that. This is what doctors do when one drug doesn't work; they just keep trying more drugs until they find one that works. Usually, they try whatever the newest research studies say is working.

Well, that new drug didn't do much for me either, and I was tired of the whole medicine game. I was tired of feeling like a guinea pig for the newest drugs out there on the market. The drugs just did not work. Every symptom I had had continued to grow worse and worse over the years, despite all of the newest and the latest drugs. Paradoxically, the asthma attacks grew worse the more asthma medication I took. Addicted to my inhalers, I couldn't breathe freely without them.

All of a sudden I developed strength of will. As a child, I had always been very passive and obedient. All of my life, I had done exactly what I was told to do - I was very very good. I had always done everything exactly the way the doctors instructed me to do it. The doctors call that being a "compliant" patient. I had always taken the shots, the pills, the syrups, the antibiotics, the antihistamines, the decongestants, the sprays, the steroids, and the inhalers without complaining. But now I made a decision - I wasn't going to do this anymore.

For the first time, I stood up to a doctor and told him I refused to take any more medicine. It was the hardest thing I ever had to do. I had no idea what would happen when I stopped it. A side effect of antidepressants are that they help the pain of migraines. The migraines had become much more bearable since I had begun the medication. Even tapering off the medication put me into a withdrawal of even worse migraines and horrifying nightmares. I had to go through that pain. I prayed and got through it. I remember flushing the rest of the medicine down the toilet, resolutely telling myself, "I'm not going to follow this road anymore."

Gradually, the bizarre hallucinations left after I discontinued the medicine. This fact seriously shook my belief in medicine. A doctor can know about side effects, but until he actually experiences them personally, he really doesn't fully understand or appreciate them. Having little understanding of how much suffering medication side effects cause makes it very easy for doctors to prescribe medications indiscriminately. Doctors who have taken a lot of these medicines seem to be more hesitant to tell people to take medicine.

As I began to take my life into my own hands, I found the strength to walk into a health food store. I was barely able to hold my self upright as I walked through the store, weak and shaking in the knees, not knowing what I would find. I finally settled on the book section. As my quivering fingers perused the pages of the books there, I realized that this place was the one last hope I had in the entire world. This was the last stop - my last chance. I told myself if I could just find information on an herb to help me with the asthma attacks that I would be happy with that. I had some glimmer of hope, and I was willing to try anything. I took several kinds of encapsulated herbs, but was very disappointed when I found that they did not help me much. I returned to the health store frequently, though, and continued to look through the book section. What did I have to lose? There had to be answers there; there was no other place to look.

At first, I was uncomfortable going to the health food store. It seemed like a hangout for hippies. Then I thought, "Why would I let such a superficial insecurity stand in the way of my healing?" – something far more important than my ego.

As time went on, I began to get more comfortable being in the health food store. One day, I noticed a book about natural methods to heal breathing problems, such as asthma and bronchitis. I didn't know personally know who the author was, but the book was not too expensive and the back cover sounded interesting. The author was a chiropractor who had a healing ranch/retreat in southern California. People with hopeless illnesses would come to this retreat and get well. The book talked about things I had never considered important like my diet, my attitude, exercise, and the importance of regular and frequent bowel movements. There were case histories in that book, one of which included the story of a woman so severely asthmatic that she could not move across the room without taking her medicine through her nebulizer. She described her healing when she changed her diet and followed the doctor's advice. I thought if that lady was that bad off, and she was able to totally heal her asthma, then I could, too.

But then my doubts began to surface. This was, after all, quackery. This was a small paperback book that came from a health food store of all places. There were no medical studies being described in this book - no *real medicine*, or so I thought. Dr. Jensen said all diseases begin in the bowel, and that most people are constipated which leads to all number of diseases. I thought, "I am not constipated; I'm regular, and this is ridiculous! Only old people have that. There must be some other reason why I'm this sick."

But this was the only book I found that said I could be well. I pondered the thought that if the cures for these diseases existed, why am I not learning them in medical school? After all, Modern Medicine had so much technology, so many medicines. We were even beginning to understand genetics and do gene splicing. How could some unknown chiropractor out in California of all places, have the answers to these diseases? It puzzled me to no end. I read it and reread it, over and over.

I began to buy other books written by the same author in hopes of understanding these new concepts and convincing myself of their validity. Fairly soon, I noticed that most of my waking hours were spent reading his books. He had written around 50 of them in all. There was plenty of time to read since I didn't have the strength to do anything else. I was obsessed with finding the answers to my questions: How had I gotten this way, and what could I do about it?

Just about everything he wrote contradicted the medicine I was learning, so I had a terrific time dealing with that. But I knew that this was my last chance, and I also knew that if something didn't change soon, that I would kill myself because I couldn't take the amount of pain I had anymore.

I knew from my reading that I was going to have to change my horrible diet of chocolates, candy bars, cookies, soft drinks, hamburgers, pizza and vending machine fare. I knew I had to walk into the produce section of the store and buy real food. At first, this terrified me. I didn't know what arugula was; I didn't know there were different kinds of cabbage. I didn't know there were all of these wonderfully nutritious forms of dark green leafy lettuces like Romaine, red leaf, green leaf, etc. All I knew about was the iceberg lettuce, which was pretty much empty of any nutrients except water and a little fiber. I bit the bullet, and decided to try one new thing each time I shopped.

And I had to teach myself how to cook. My idea of cooking was throwing something frozen into the microwave. I became an expert on how to make stir-fry with vegetables and brown rice. I ate an apple a day in hopes that it would keep the doctors away. Really! I bought lots of healthy cookbooks and tried the best I could. The new rule was that if I cooked something, no matter how it tasted, I had to eat it. And I always followed the rule because I was very motivated and I knew my life depended on it. Gradually, my taste buds adapted to the taste of real food, and I found myself actually enjoying the learning experience. I began to enjoy spelt pasta and quinoa cereal with things like soy milk and almond milk. I had forgotten what real food tasted like since for most of my life I had always eaten processed foods- things made with all-purpose flour, sugar, salt - things that came in a can or a box or a bag. I discovered the joy of spices - curries, dill, marinades, etc. I learned what tofu was and how to make it taste good. I started to feel stronger. Something was happening.

At that point, I did an even stranger thing; I began discussing these new healing concepts with my psychiatrist. I told him all about the author's assertions that no matter what the problem is, it can be fixed with nutrition and other changes in lifestyle. I told him about how when you feed the body the proper nutrients, it begins to gradually gather enough strength to throw off poisons that have accumulated there from living an unhealthy life full of chemicals, preservatives, pollution, and being constipated. I had already stopped drinking any alcoholic beverages, had stopped eating anything with refined sugar in it, and had become an unwilling vegetarian.

He did not seem too impressed, and thought that I might be becoming too obsessed with my food intake. Since I was so thin, it was easy for him to consider me a mental case and now an anorexic one. He wasn't aware of the fact that I was quite known for eating large amounts of food and yet I continued to lose weight. The problem was a severe hyperthyroidism that caused the extreme weakness, heart arrhythmias, and the episodes at night. But his job was not to evaluate me physically - it was to pick apart my brain and label it as wrong. He was looking for me to have mental disorders because that's what he knew how to diagnose.

But at the time, I was desperate and wanted answers. I wanted an action plan. He didn't have an action plan. We didn't discuss healing options that would empower me. I was much too ill to understand this was not the right doctor to visit to get well. He felt it necessary to repeatedly remind me that it was *PANIC DISORDER* I had, not a physical condition. Nothing I said convinced him otherwise. He reiterated several times that I was unable to deal with having a mental disorder, therefore, I had made myself to believe that I had a physical disease instead. Actually, it was the reverse.

He brought out the psychiatric manual, and referred to the symptoms of panic disorder as matching my own. I told him those symptoms could be caused by many things, not just by panic disorder. Much later on, I found these symptoms were all caused by having epileptic seizures and hyperthyroidism.

At that time, I felt completely powerless because by now I finally realized that I had a severe problem, yet no doctor would believe me. I knew the psychiatrist cared, and that meant something to me. He really believed that he was right, and I knew that he was trying to help me in his own way - but luckily for me, I tired of these weekly unproductive sessions. He didn't know any more about nutrition than did the average American, and that wasn't much. He didn't look all that healthy, either.

It was not a matter of finding the right doctor. It was a matter of listening to the one doctor inside - my inner voice that had been trying to tell me many things about myself for years. Yet, I had not been willing to listen to that inner wisdom, because I had already willingly given all of that power away to the doctors - after all, they were the experts on these matters.

My inner wisdom kept trying to tell me that something was drastically wrong that needed my immediate attention. I kept holding out for miracle drugs. Medicine would save the day. I was spending thousands of dollars learning a system scientifically advanced of medicine that saved millions of lives. Medicine would save the day with an easy diagnosis and an easy pill, and I wouldn't have to take very much responsibility at all for making changes to a life that wasn't working. This is what I believed.

Around this time, two events happened that finally broke through all of my denial and changed everything. The first was that one evening I had a massive episode of chest pain. The pain was so bad this time that I could not move. I lay on my back on the floor and was unable to do anything except try to breathe. I lay there struggling to inhale and exhale only a few feet away from the phone. *Oh my God! Am I going to die? Is this it?* I thought maybe this would be a good time to call an ambulance. I was only able to slowly drag my body inch by inch to the phone. *No! Not now!* I prayed, *No! Not yet!* After what seemed to be an eternity, my fingers touched the foot of the file cabinet. *Thank you, God!* I hoisted myself up alongside the small cabinet. Desperately clinging to it, I attempted to reach the phone. After a few half-hearted and badly aimed attempts, I actually was able to pick up the phone. *Please, not yet!*, I begged.

By this time, the pain had made me delirious. But, there at the phone, I made a decision. I already knew what ambulances and emergency rooms were like. I figured I'd be waiting all night to be seen, and by the time someone saw me, they'd look in my medical chart like so many times before, see that panic disorder there, and not do anything to help me anyway. I couldn't stand to die that way in the middle of a chaotic emergency room filled with the horrid sounds of pain and screaming. If I was going to die, I wanted to die peacefully at home.

The decision was to <u>not</u> call 9-1-1. Those three simple numbers would've brought help to me, but right then, I decided I did not want that kind of help anymore. No more pills, no more doctors, no more diagnoses, no more pain. No more sterile, detached clinical judgments. I only wanted release from this horrible nightmare that I had lived for the past two years. I clumsily set down the receiver, missed several times and fell straight to the floor again to remain in that spot the rest of the night. Every last bit of my energy had been spent just getting to the phone.

I was too tired to continue breathing and wondered how long I would hold out. I began to pray again, but in a different way. I explained to God that I was finally ready to accept whatever was about to happen. The odd thing about it is that I didn't consider myself to be particularly religious at that point of my life; I didn't even go to church. As I had been *raised* Catholic, though, I <u>knew</u> I had to confess all of my sins to God. According to Catholic belief, if all of your sins are not confessed and you die, you will go to purgatory where you will suffer more before you finally get to heaven. I didn't want to go to purgatory after this experience.

I told God I was sorry for every wrong thing, every wrong thought and every wrong deed that I had ever committed, and I thanked Him for providing me with the amount of time I had lived on this earth. Unable to speak, I silently prayed in my head every Catholic prayer that I had ever learned, even ones that I thought I had forgotten. I prayed that my family would not find my possessions too much of a burden, and I wondered how they would take the news of my death. Most of all, I prayed for God to be with me to help me bear the pain. I lay there on my back on the floor for several hours unable to move, and my life literally flashed before my eyes - the good, the bad, the ecstatic moments, as well as the painful ones. Time stood still while my mind raced at what seemed like the speed of light through the important and even the trivial parts of my life. What had it meant, this life of mine? Was it worth it? Had it been completed?

The happy moments came up - I had always been a thrill seeker. Since childhood I would ride any rollercoaster. I delighted in the sensation of my stomach rising and falling with the rollercoaster and the wind furiously whipping through my hair. We used to stand up in our seats and hold our arms up. As children, my brothers and I would build snow forts complete with an ice sheet as the ceiling and have snow-ball fights; we were merciless; we threw hard. I would smack the heck out of a tennis ball just for the pure joy of knowing I was able to hit it that hard...Now everything was abruptly coming to an end.

In my childhood, I was a swimmer and a tennis player. In my teenage years, I had been a runner for both the track and cross-country teams - the thrill of competition excited me. Once I even won a race - I remember the feel of the tape across my chest as I crossed the finish line in a sprint, trying to beat the other competitor next to me. I was fiercely proud of that. Running always made me feel so free - nothing could slow me down.

In my youth I was unstoppable. I went bungy jumping off of a bridge in New Zealand in the middle of winter over the top of a frozen river. I went snorkeling along the Great Barrier Reef. There was nothing I wouldn't do. Just after college, my boyfriend told me I wouldn't dare do a tequila shot that contained a worm - "shooting the worm," they called it.

I "shot the worm" and grinned at him while he sat there amazed that I had done it because "You're a girl," he said.

I delighted in shocking people with my fearlessness. I adored heights and would go to the tops of many a building and lean over the railing. I indulged my love of heights when I became a college cheerleader. Since I was the lightest, they would put me on top of the pyramids. I shot to the top with not the least bit of fear.

I took boat rides and cruises, trains and trolleys, trying to explore and conquer the world around me. I had traipsed around Europe and toured Paris, sometimes on my own - there were no barriers holding me back then. The beauty of Paris was something I could never forget. I stood before the magnificence of the Grand Canyon and Mount Rushmore and watched with awe while the geysers went off at Yellowstone

National Park.

I prayed again, "God, if this is your will for me to die, I will let go, but if I am to survive this, I'm not going to tolerate this pain anymore!" Suddenly, a sense of perfect peace swept through every cell in my body. I felt totally enveloped by a warm blanket of indescribable love, and knew that it was safe to let go. No longer afraid, I finally allowed my eyes to close, and nothing at all mattered anymore about my life. My studies, my friends, my parents, my clothes, my furniture, my possessions -- even my identity were all completely unimportant. I felt a part of everything, and everything a part of me, and it was the most blissful experience I had ever had. I realized that God had been loving me and caring for me all of my life. I saw the folly of my anger and irritations, and the worry I had carried around me all of my years. For the first time in my life, I felt God and *knew* that He was real.

I thought I must have been dead when I first awoke the next morning. Somehow, the pain had disappeared. Was I in heaven? After a few minutes, though, I abruptly realized that I was actually still alive. There I was still on the floor by the phone. I figured God must really want me alive if I'm still here after all of that! The pain was temporarily gone, but nothing else had changed. I thought maybe I must have been crazy to think that I was dying because I obviously had not. Amazingly, life just went on. Utterly exhausted, I slept all day, unable to shake off the experience, though, and I had no idea the impact this experience would have on the rest of my life.

A few days later, I was lying on the floor of my apartment right after a seizure, but still did not know that I had had one. The phone rang, and I grabbed the receiver without really knowing what I had. A very good friend of mine was on the other end. For some reason, I could not figure out where that sound was coming from. I didn't know if it was the doorbell, the phone, the alarm clock or the television. The noise was the sound of my friend's voice. I tried to ask where the sound was coming from, but only gibberish left my lips. I called my friend the wrong name, and then started speaking nonsense, unable to put even two words together. He kept asking me what was I saying? More gibberish spewed out of my mouth.

All at once, I understood I was on the phone with the guy who had sat behind me in class every day for two years, and I screamed at him, "How do you expect me to know what's going on; I'm hypoglycemic!" That was the last straw. When I realized I couldn't even speak, I knew something was really seriously wrong. I couldn't deny it anymore!

Now lucid, I hung up, and immediately grabbed the phone book, scouring the yellow pages for a nutritionist, like the author of the breathing book. I knew I could not do it alone anymore. My only requirement as I scanned the pages was that the person was not an MD. No more doctors. No more medicine! I chose never to return to the psychiatrist. I know now that I couldn't allow anyone or anything to stand in the way of my healing.

Letting Go of Medicine

Very briefly, I talked with the nutritionist on the phone and asked if she did any Glucose Tolerance Tests to test for hypoglycemia (a condition where the level of sugar in the blood is too low). She told me that that test was irrelevant to my condition, and that she would explain why when I got there. I felt a great sense of relief as she seemed to know exactly what she was talking about. *Maybe it's something simple*, I hoped.

C H A P T E R 7

A New Beginning

The Adjustment

Well, thank God that it was summertime and I had a couple of months off in order to adjust to the gigantic change in lifestyle I was about to make. There was no doubt that the changes I had implemented from my readings at the health food store had carried me this far. But there was so much more to do to get myself well.

I still remember it like it was yesterday - the hopes and expectations I felt as I drove up to a quaint old house in the middle of town. Would this lady be able to help me? Was there any hope at all? Was I going to survive this? The sign for the nutritionist's clinic was not very prominent, and I think I passed it three times before I finally found the place. I walked inside, in search of clues as to what kind of person she was going to be.

No one was at the reception area which I thought was odd, but I knew that this was no ordinary place. I tentatively rang the little bell, as if ringing it louder would be too much of an intrusion, before I finally came to rest on a plush sofa in front of a fireplace. I was so tense and uncertain about it all, I think I would have jumped if a pin had dropped. Finally, my name was called and I was told to spit and pee in two separate cups. This would later become a weekly ritual. They were to be analyzed using Ream's Method, and those tests would tell me how I was progressing.

I sat in a chair facing her desk, and listened as Claire explained the physical mechanics behind why I was sick. She told me my adrenal glands were exhausted, and that I could not get well until they were healed. She said it would probably take about four months. I also had Candida yeast overgrowing in my system causing all sorts of problems.

I was given two books to look through describing the "Program" and she told me she'd have more information after the hair analysis came back. Wait - hair analysis? She told me that I was toxic in the large intestine and that I would be doing coffee enemas daily to cleanse my bowel, and colonics once a week. Enemas? I didn't even know how to do one. And what's a colonic? She told me I needed to drink my carrot juice fresh instead of the frozen kind I had been drinking. What? You mean I have to use a juicer every day? Then she proceeded to go down a long list of supplements (4 pages to be exact) checking off all of the supplements I would need to take. The program would be especially designed for my particular metabolism.

She told me that the two worst foods on the planet were dairy products and wheat, and that these caused more problems than anything else. I asked, "Why?" She answered that when people eliminated these from their diets, they got dramatic healing results.

Then there were two pages telling me *exactly* what I could and what I couldn't eat. No red meat, no animal fat or blood, nothing fried, no alcohol, no refined sugar, no salt, no MSG (monosodium glutamate), no sweets, no dairy products, no tomatoes, no wheat, no soft drinks, coffee, tea or chocolate, and the list went on. In addition, I had to drink at least 20 ounces of carrot juice every day mixed with beet juice, celery juice and the juices of other greens. This combination was building up my blood. I would need to take a barley grass mixture, beta carotene, Coenzyme Q10, digestive enzymes, antioxidants, aloe vera juice concentrate, food grade hydrogen peroxide, calcium and magnesium, lots of potassium, an acidophilus powder, homeopathic preparations, herbal tinctures, borage oil, and take 4 ounces of fresh lemon juice squeezed into 28 ounces of distilled water daily, and that was only the beginning. *Oh my God!*

It was an initiation of sorts, as I learned all kinds of things and was being introduced all at once to this huge program that I was about to undertake. Her assistant Joanne took me upstairs into the adjoining health food store and explained the details to me, as well as answering any questions I had. She worked there with Claire in large part because she herself had been healed by going through the program. I only halfway understood her because I was so ill that I couldn't concentrate on what she was saying long enough for her to finish a sentence. But, she clipped some of my hair from an inconspicuous place on my scalp and put it in an envelope to be sent to an institute out of state for analysis. Later on, my hairdresser found that spot and threw a fit about it. I just didn't have the guts to tell him that I had gotten a "hair analysis."

I walked out of that health food store with a huge grocery bag filled with supplements that I could barely carry, and figured that I had spent hundreds of dollars that day. It didn't really matter, though, since I figured I was going to die anyway.

All of the patients there lovingly referred to it as "the Program." I saw many of them in the waiting room as I went for a recheck every week. We commonly discussed what had brought us there and what kind of results we were getting. I slowly built myself a support system out of the nutritionist's office staff and fellow patients. These were the only people who I could truly relate to and who could truly relate to me. None of them ever told me I was doing the wrong thing or that I needed to see a *real* doctor. They were the ones who had already *been* to the *real* doctors numerous times, and had been given up on, and told they were hopeless and incurable. Many times, they were told they only had a few weeks or months to live.

We were the only ones who knew that a total healing was possible. We were the only ones who knew what this program was all about. All of the patients told me that the reason they came was because a friend or relative of theirs had come previously and had been healed of some incurable condition - things like breast cancer, colon and rectal cancer, arthritis, lupus, lung cancer, pancreatic cancer, thyroid cancer, migraines, parasites, Lou Gehrig's disease, brain tumors, and many other diseases. I was the only one who came because of the Yellow Pages. (I supposed I lucked out by *not* picking an MD.) She didn't need to advertise; her clinic was full and booming because people got healed, and when they were healed, they spread the word like wildfire.

These were all diseases that I knew from my schooling to be incurable, of course. What I saw healed there was beyond my wildest expectations. Nothing in my life up until this point had prepared me for this. Nothing in my first two years of medical school had prepared me for this. People were healing right before my very eyes. There went my disbelief and my scientific need to prove everything.

I realized at that point that medical science knew hardly anything at all about how the human body works, why it breaks down into disease, or about the potential it has to completely heal and repair itself. It wasn't until I actually saw the miracles first hand, and so many of them, that I very first became a believer. I had always been a skeptic and a doubter of everything. I wanted to see proof. There it was sitting right across from me as the lady told me about how the arthritis almost destroyed her hip. The doctor told her she'd be in a wheelchair the rest of her life with a hip replacement, and now, her hip was totally rebuilt just by her dietary changes, nutritional supplements, and her faith.

I had to change everything, especially my taste buds. The first time I tasted carrot juice, it was from a can. I swore I'd never drink that gross stuff again. The next time, I had it thawed out from being frozen. That was a little better. When I juiced it fresh, it was much better, but when I mixed it with the beets and other greens, it began to take on a hue somewhat reminiscent of dark venous blood. Being a doctor-in-training, it bothered me to be drinking something that looked like blood - I saw plenty of that during my medical training. I used to pretend that I was Count Dracula and this was my "blood cocktail." I had to make it funny somehow - this program was tough! But, each time I was in the clinic, I heard stories about how so many cancers had been healed with carrot juice. It was ascribed magical, miraculous healing powers, and I still know it to be true today.

I flat out had to hold my nose to get the aloe concentrate down - that's one of the nastiest tasting substances I've ever had. I found the trick to that was *not* to exhale until several seconds after it was all down. However, I did all of the program exactly as it was listed. I didn't pick and choose as I heard some of the other patients did, as I was beginning to have hope now: I could see the possibility of my own healing. I wanted to fight so I could live.

Most importantly, what I had to learn was how to get a better attitude - the proper attitude for healing. I couldn't just approach my healing as horrible tasting concoctions, and the inconvenience of making myself fresh juice every day. I could have given myself a hundred reasons why I didn't like this program, but the fact of the matter was that it was MY program and it was doing for me what I put into it. I had to drink that juice and be thankful that it was healing me. I had to learn to sing in the kitchen and not mind the extra cleanup because I prepared food fresh instead of getting fast food through the drive-through which I used to do quite frequently. I had to have the attitude that while enemas and colonics may not be cool, they were getting toxic poisons out of my body and therefore a wonderful and valuable healing tool. I had to look at the expense as something I was glad to spend money on because I was worth it.

I couldn't afford this program, but that did not stop me. I wanted to live, so I borrowed money. Eventually, I sold many of my possessions. Again, I wanted to live. I was not going to die from a flimsy excuse I made up not to get well. Finally, I had to look at the whole experience as something that somehow was benefiting me, and that I was experiencing life exactly the way I was supposed to be every minute of the day.

There were so many things to do that I literally had to make lists and refer to them frequently in order to remember exactly what to take and when. There were so many capsules to take that I used to take around 25 of them at a time. No wonder my esophagus would go into spasms. But I found a way to deal with all that, (anyone who *really* wants to, does), and pretty soon, I was popping those supplements down like a pro. I was too embarrassed to tell many people that I was putting forth this much effort and that much money to get well when the only official diagnosis I had gotten from a medical doctor was a mental disorder. I was afraid people would think I had gone nuts, that I was gullible, and that I was wasting my money.

There were days I had the energy to make the carrot juice, but not the strength to drink it. Many times, I would fall asleep right in the middle of drinking it. I would wake up in the middle of the night with old, stale carrot juice, wondering whether or not I should drink it. But, I didn't give up. I just kept telling myself, that tomorrow, I'd be able to drink a little more. It was not easy. But, I know now that God carried me through it.

There was a long flight of stairs that led up to Claire's health food store. I prayed for the ability to make each step, grabbed onto the handrail and dragged myself up with fierce determination. Now I was fighting; there was hope and I was not going to quit. I would force myself to carry all of the food and supplements I bought down the stairs by myself. I remember many days where every step was agonizing. I wouldn't let anyone help me - I refused to think of myself as that sick. I would always be able to carry my own groceries!

The amazing thing about this program was that it was working. As an act of faith, the day before my first appointment, I threw out all of my asthma inhalers. The medical doctors would've gone nuts about that. I didn't care about what the doctors believed anymore. They had their chance. Now, *I was having mine.* So, the asthma improved solely I think because I stopped taking the inhalers. I still had asthma attacks for a while, but they were not as severe, and I flat out refused to take the medicines anymore. In fact, I refused to identify myself as an asthmatic anymore. I never took an inhaler ever again. I slowly began to gain more strength, and to have less headaches or any of the other pains.

I stopped my allergy shots for the first time since I was a child and decided not to take them ever again. I threw the allergy shot medication away. I realized the folly of the chemicals in my refrigerator. After all, how was I going to get a healing from medication that might give me an allergic reaction so severe, I might require a shot of adrenaline to block it? It did not seem logical to me. I don't know why I had never in my life made this realization before because it was very obvious to me at this point.

So, by the time I got to the Nutritionist's office, and she asked me what medications I was on, I told her, "Nothing... anymore." And she said, "Good." It was much easier for her to work with conditions which weren't complicated by the use of medications. The use of medications made it twice as hard to heal a disease.

If it was a miracle to see these people and myself getting well, it was seriously a miracle to see **exactly how** this happened. This was **not** something called a spontaneous remission. This was people doing a lot of work, making changes, putting healing substances into their bodies, and changing their lives. It was a process called detoxification. In other words, poisons that had accumulated in my body over the years were being released into the bloodstream and into the large intestine for removal. The poisons came in many different varieties and were too numerous to name, so we just called them "toxins." What were they? Chemicals, pesticides, herbicides, household cleaners, food additives, preservatives, heavy metals, paint fumes, gasoline fumes, intestinal and liver parasites; in short, toxins accumulated from being exposed to a modern, industrialized chemically-laden way of life. The modern way of living put people's adrenal glands under too much stress and exhausted them, slowing down the metabolism, thus slowing down the body's ability to process and filter out these environmental contaminants. We learned that the toxins were stored in the liver and that this deranged the metabolism, leaving the body unprotected and open to all sorts of diseases. I say "we" because all of us patients learned together and supported each other. Imagine - a doctor learning about healing instead of about disease. And I was learning not as a doctor, but as a patient, along with other patients. These people were the only support I had.

We found out that a detoxification was a period of time during which the body all of a sudden let go of these toxins, which meant that a person felt badly during this time - there were toxic chemicals released into the bloodstream that previously had been stored away in muscle cells, fat cells, bone cells, the liver, etc. During this time, any symptom from the past could be re-experienced, sometimes in a more intense way as the toxins worked themselves out of the body. The process was helped along by the many enemas and colonics as they drew the toxins out faster and thus relieved many of the detoxification symptoms. For me, this included headaches, migraines, joint pains, asthma attacks, and many other strange things. But these were not disease symptoms; these were the good symptoms of healing. It was strange at first because it felt like I had made myself sicker. But I knew that this was the process one had to go through, and that other people had gone through to get well. So, I was patient. I was very patient. After the symptoms abated, I would find myself stronger and healthier, and this was exactly the way it was supposed to happen. I was right on schedule.

Sometimes, in the middle of a detoxification I would just feel like crying forever. Maybe it was because it meant that I was back on the floor again unable to get up, and that was very frustrating for me, but I also knew that not only were old toxic chemicals being released from my body, but also old emotions that had been stuck in my body and never released. So, I just cried and let them out. Through these emotional healing crises, I gradually realized how I had made myself ill with my hatred, my judgments, my unwillingness to let go and forgive, my perfectionism, and my insecurities. I learned to pay attention to my symptoms, and I dared to listen to the answers my body gave me about why it was all happening. No doctor in the world could have told me why I was sick except for the real doctor inside me - the real doctor that lies in all of us. I realized a direct connection between the way I had been living and the way I was feeling now.

The process was, in a very personal way, the direct consequence of living out of balance with nature. I really *felt* the damaging effects of all the candy bars I had eaten. I felt the effect of the pies and cakes and cookies and doughnuts that I had eaten all those years with the wrong assumption that they would do me no harm. I developed an appreciation for the miracle that happens when the body overthrows toxic, weak tissue and chemicals and forces them out. I had been suffering all those years from "sins of the flesh." I had violated the laws of nature, and I had paid the price with my ill health. My body had been trying to survive despite all of the abuse I had given it. Despite my ill treatment of it, my body was very forgiving and wanted to give me another chance. Recognizing this, I never wanted to eat those chocolate candies again, and I never have.

The big surprise was that I had parasites. Claire was not at all surprised. She told me that anyone with a serious disease and every single patient with cancer she had ever seen had parasites. So, I passed a few bowlfuls of what looked like intestinal flukes. It was pretty scary, but it was painless and they looked dead. As I described them to Claire, she remarked, "Oh, yeah, *those*. Those are very common. I used to send off samples to Mexico for identification. They'll send you pages of information on what kind it is, what symptoms it causes, and information about the whole life cycle - everything you wanted to know and things that you don't. I had to send them to Mexico because every time I sent one of my patients to get a parasite test in America, it always turned out negative, and then they would pass a great big tapeworm or other parasites. I had to find out what they were."

She was always very direct, which was one of the qualities in her that I really admired. Her directness, I could only guess, came from her long experience of taking people through hopeless situations and getting them past their belief that they were hopeless and that nothing could be done. Claire's confidence in the Program was unshakable. She had to be that strong to make up for her patients' weaknesses.

I had another routine checkup with the family doctor at that time. Many people might not understand why I went back to the doctor at all. But there was still my scientific curiosity that would get the best of me, and I'd think, "Oh, maybe now the doctors can diagnose what's really wrong." Little did I know at that time that **getting healed has nothing to do with what your particular diagnosis is** - those details are just not important in natural healing. I kept going to my family doctor because I knew he really cared. I also knew the psychiatrist cared and that's why I continued to see him for a while. It's just that they had no idea how to heal me. So, when I told him about the bowlfuls of parasites, the family doctor quipped, "People don't just pass parasites." I already knew that's what they were; I was furious that he didn't believe me. This was true! I knew from what was happening at the clinic that everybody who was seriously ill had passed or was presently passing parasites, and when they passed them, their health took a dramatic turn for the better. I don't like to argue, so I got up and left without pressing the matter. So what. It's not his fault he didn't know anything about natural healing.

I guess I expected the doctor to believe me because it was true. No, it doesn't happen that way. He expected randomized, double-blinded, multi-center trial research studies showing it to be true before he would accept it as fact.

Detoxifying was work, and I wanted to give up many times, only I wouldn't let myself. I would find another natural healing book and read it. I'd read ones I'd already read over and over again. Edward, in his generosity, had given me a cassette tape with several songs on it, one of which was called "Don't Give Up." I remember playing that song over and over and over, trying to motivate myself to continue. I was not going to give up. I was not a quitter. The chiropractor wrote in his book that anyone could be healed, and I was going to have my healing no matter what.

As the heavy metals came out, I would experience the taste of metal in my mouth. "Oh, yes," Claire would say, "Anyone who's toxic with metals has that." Charlene and I used to joke about it feeling like there was a penny always in our mouths. I had that for several months, as my body unloaded all of that toxic material. What was it? Claire would tell me that the most common was aluminum, then copper, then mercury, and lastly, lead. The lead, though, was so toxic, that the body wouldn't let go of it for at least 2 years, not until the body was so strong and healthy that it could stand the release of something so highly toxic into the bloodstream and finally out of the body. She told me that many times she would do a hair analysis on a person during these times, and she would see an elevated lab value of the particular metal being eliminated.

I always wondered if there was a blood test that would measure these metals in the blood because I knew if there were, mine would be positive for them. I would have that metal taste in my mouth for months and months while I unloaded what felt like tons of heavy metals from my body, and as I did so, I felt slowly better and better. I was shocked at the amount of junk in my body that wasn't supposed to be there. No wonder I was so ill!

Charlene worked at the health food store. She worked there because she had gotten dramatic results ridding herself of lupus, and was still was there doing the Program five years later. It was the only way she felt good. She was the sweetest, most empathetic person I had ever met. Knowing her was a blessing and gave me more courage to go on. We talked for hours about the Program, and what was going on in our lives. She became my very good friend. One of our favorite topics of conversation was about how someone termed incurable would go back to the doctor after having done the Program, and the doctor would say they had a spontaneous remission. We called the clinic the place of spontaneous remissions because almost everyone who did the Program got one. We knew it was a detoxification.

I remember talking to her sometimes, and she would be in the middle of a cleansing reaction where she'd break out in a rash from the lupus in the past, and she'd tell me she felt like shit. I'd tell her I felt like shit, too, and it was a funny way of bonding, but we talked real and openly about what was happening to all of us.

I began to look forward to my weekly visits, as I was felt so much emotional support there. We learned what to say about the program so that it didn't scare people so much. Some patients' spouses didn't even know about obvious parts of the Program. Everyone was embarrassed about the enemas and colonics, but Claire's face never showed a trace of embarrassment. She was emphatic about their importance. Intestinal toxins contributed to and caused every disease. There were stories of her chasing down sick people threatening to plug them into a colonic and give them a good cleaning. Obviously, the stories were more rumor than fact, but they always allowed for a much needed belly laugh.

Claire was a master at showing the right facial expression to convey emphasis when needed. She knew exactly how to give that look of disapproval when someone didn't do all the parts of the Program. That was all that I needed to try even harder for the next week. Sometimes I even heard fights going on from the waiting room. I knew how much Claire loved her patients. I knew that she was trying to get them out of their pitiful excuses for not doing the Program, for not getting well.

You'd think that everyone would want to get well. However, this is not the case. When people don't want to get well, they make up all sorts of excuses for not following the health program and search for ways to prove that the program doesn't work. They even find fault with the healer, even though they have received dramatic results. Some would dare call it quackery because they knew **that** accusation would get to her. Sometimes the brainwashing that diseases are incurable from the medical profession is so strong that many patients can't even admit when they're healed that they're actually **healed**. They consider it a fluke - an accident that they got well. She won some; she lost some.

Once, just after an argument with Claire, a patient yelled at me, "Have you ever had any problems with Claire?!" Her face was red, nostrils were flaring, and I wouldn't give her any ammunition at all. I knew you had to make changes if you wanted to get well. Change is not easy. We all want to fight the changes, so we get angry at whatever is pushing us to change. There were many things about my Program that I disagreed with. There were many times I was angry, but I absolutely could not deny the fact that I was healing. Nothing else was important. Everything else was minor details.

Then out came more toxins: this time, old antibiotics came out in my urine, and I hadn't taken any antibiotics in over a year. I remember the horrible, distinctive smell of those antibiotics, the first time on the way in, and the second time on the way out of my body. Of course, Claire had a great story to illustrate the point that chemical drugs leave residues in the body. The body cannot all the way process them out, but during a detoxification, it all comes out. She told me a story about a woman who had taken one steroid pill and her abdomen blew up like a balloon. She evidently was in this state for months until she came to Claire. After doing the Program, the pill came out, and her colon went all the way down again. Claire always had a great story. In fact, while I was at the clinic, frequently, previous patients of hers would come by to say hello and that they were still doing fine. These were always very happy occasions. There was smiling and laughing and kissing, and emotional expressions of gratitude. In fact, her office was littered with letters and postcards expressing these sentiments. This was like no doctor's office I had ever visited before.

"Your liver is one of the most toxic I've ever seen," Claire would tell me, as the detoxification process in me seemed to be so intense and so prolonged. It became evident during this process that I was much sicker than when I had told her I thought the problem was that I was hypoglycemic. "The most toxic one I ever saw was in a lady who was a heroin addict." I was disappointed - I didn't even get the pain-relieving benefits of the heroin to get my liver so toxic. I believe it must have been all of those over-the-counter pain relievers.

Over the next year and a half that I was on that Program, my brain began to rebuild itself. It goes without saying that I had damaged it from having so many seizures. I later estimated that I had had one every day and every night for a couple of years without knowing it. But my brain began to rebuild, and the way this occurred over time was that I would spontaneously have memories come up from the past. They came up from the near past and from the far past. Some were pleasant, some were neutral, and some were unpleasant. But I began to realize over time, that new neural connections were being reestablished, and that my brain was healing. No one prepared me for this, although it wouldn't have changed what I did.

It was a wondrous experience. I began to remember who I was based on my past that I was slowly beginning to recall. I soon felt like a real person with a real identity again. It was such a blessing. After several months, I realized that I could think and concentrate better, and that I could hold longer conversations with people. I remember watching the movie *Awakenings*, and saying to myself, "That's me! I'm waking up!"

Ironically, at the same time I was regenerating my brain, I was learning in medical school that brain cells do not regenerate. Somehow, I did not believe them.

Doing this program gave me the strength to go on to what's considered the most grueling year of medical school -

the third year. The vacation was officially over. Now, there was another huge adjustment to make: going back to school with the knowledge of natural healing. This would be an even harder adjustment than the first one. I knew too much. I couldn't just forget everything I had seen and experienced. So, I questioned all of the medical theories and I didn't buy into them. By the end of the summer, I had finally realized what an incredible miracle it was that I was still alive. *Maybe I won't die after all.*

The Shock of the Clinical Years

I began the third year of my training, the "clinical years" they were called, putting all of that classroom knowledge to use by seeing patients in the hospital and in clinics - interviewing them, examining them, and helping to determine their treatment plan. The year was blocked into 6-week long rotations. Many were required, like the basic OBGYN, family practice, internal medicine, surgery, and for others, we had some choice in the matter.

Since I had begun to see the horrors of what modern medicine can create, I hated my time working in the hospital. My peers liked it, I assumed, although for them the rigorous training manifested itself in fatigue and frequent illnesses. I later met a resident who had chronic sinus problems. The doctors did a surgery on her sinuses to create a larger opening for them to drain better. After the surgery, she was still having the problem.

It was difficult at times to justify our mistreatment because we were actually paying money to see patients. We were paying a lot of money to have this hellish physically and emotionally demanding experience. It's considered the hardest year of medical school - staying up all night on call, working ungodly hours, and unending responsibilities. To undertake something like this in my condition was nothing short of crazy, but at that point, I had no idea how strenuous or how difficult it would be. I still wasn't even aware of what exactly was wrong with me or how serious it was.

During this time, I discovered how Western Medicine

encourages people to continue their bad health habits - how it keeps people victims. People didn't mind not caring for their bodies because all they had to do was go to the doctor, get some medication and the problem would be fixed - at least temporarily, and besides, insurance paid for it. There were no incentives for not smoking, or for eating a healthy diet, or for exercising. When the HMO's came along, it got worse, because then people were only paying a $10 or $15 co-pay for a doctor visit. I saw diabetics continue their candy-eating, cola-drinking lifestyles because they had been told that it was an incurable disease anyway and that nothing could be done. Because the insulin would temporarily fix the blood sugar level, these people ate anything they wanted, and consequently, over the years, required more and more insulin and more and more intervention by the doctors - things like laser surgery for the eye problems, coronary bypass surgeries, amputations, dialysis, and more and more medications.

I watched people accept this "victim" role willingly, while they listened to the latest research that showed it wasn't their fault at all - it was a faulty gene they had inherited. I watched people die of their horrible diets (everyone), their horrible work hours (the heart patients), their horrible attitudes (the diabetics and the heart patients), their horrible exercise routine and their smoking and drinking habits (the cancer, hepatitis, cirrhosis, pancreatitis, pneumonia and collapsed lung patients.) But rarely did I ever see someone die or be ill because of a faulty gene. I saw people "cop out." They figured nothing could be done, so they hoped like the rest of the American public that someday someone would find a "cure" for their supposed genetic disorder - things like obesity, diabetes, cystic fibrosis, breast cancer, colon cancer, etc. But meanwhile, they might as well drink their beer and eat their cholesterol-and fat-filled sausage and pepperoni pizza with ice cream for dessert.

So people believed – just as I had previously - that their disease was just bad luck instead of being caused by their bad living habits. Although everyone thought they were living pretty much healthy, they had no idea that the chemicals in their homes and workplace and in their foods were killing them, and they had no idea that they could be healed.

Every time I saw a patient, I wanted to tell them that they could heal themselves, if they chose to go to the natural healing clinic. But, I couldn't. I wasn't allowed to mention such things. Such things were not scientifically proven. I watched them die out of ignorance while I sat by unable to do anything but take more lab tests and report back to my attending physicians. Their cries reached out and grabbed my heart. Their screams devastated me. I knew it was unnecessary. I knew they did not have to suffer or die that way. All I could do was sneak as many as I could information about how to heal themselves naturally, and hope that they wouldn't tell their doctors. That would be serious trouble for me. So, I made them swear not to tell their doctors what I had told them, and told them that if they did, the doctors would say they were crazy. That would have been the truth.

Half of them never followed my advice because they were never convinced that they could be healed. Just as I had been, they had been brainwashed over the years that when the doctor says that's all that can be done, that's all that can be done. Period. I cried. I wanted to help every one of them, but the system was not allowing me to do anything.

Because of the horrible things I saw, I began to lead a double life. I came to the hospital, smiled and did everything the professors said. Then I would go to the natural healing clinic, share my disgust at what was going on at the hospital, as compared to the healings happening there. I don't know why I continued my training, but a big factor was the fact that I had already borrowed $40,000 to pay for this supposedly top rate medical training, and I had no way to pay it off if I quit. I was stuck, and my parents didn't have that kind of money. And I didn't know what else to do with my life.

In the beginning, I would try to test the waters with my friends. I would tell them a little bit about the healing program I was on. Sometimes, I would share a little with the residents in training. Every once in a while, a professor would ask about the funny things I did.

The funny things I did. Well, the only way I could continue the Program and go to the hospital every day was to carry everything with me. I carried around a back pack filled with lemon water, distilled water, and bottles of supplements. I packed my own lunch as I refused to eat the overly processed, nutritionally depleted food that was served in the hospital. No wonder the patients took so long to recover.

People always wanted to know why was I doing that? As I began to explain though, the reception was less than ideal. My really close friends said nothing. I supposed they didn't want to hurt my feelings. My fellow students were convinced I was seeing a quack, and that I should see a "real" doctor immediately

They were quite blunt about what they thought I should do. Because of this, I began to talk in a very vague way about it, eventually to the point where, by the end of the year, hardly anyone knew anything at all about what I was doing. It was rather strange to have friends in medical school, yet I could not share my real feelings with them - those beliefs were considered dangerous and heretical. I didn't want to explain it anymore, only to have someone tell me how wrong I was about it, and that I was doing the wrong thing - all I needed to do was find the right doctor, they said. I once believed that to be true, but I didn't fall for that anymore. I had already been to all of the doctors.

I remember during my second year, there were professors who gave lectures on how dangerous alternative medicine is. They would show slides of alternative medicine gone wrong. They told us how a man almost died from a serious bacterial infection that came from the rattlesnake capsules he got from a local natural healer. Nobody at Claire's clinic took rattlesnake capsules. They lectured to us about how moxibustion can cause severe burns. The slides they showed were shocking, and my friends had these stark images branded into their minds that alternative medicine is dangerous. It would never occur to them that the material being lectured about was an extremely small segment of alternative medicine.

There are quacks everywhere. But, it is now my belief that most of them belong to the medical profession. When chemical medicine first came into existence in the 1940's, the prevailing belief at that time was that these doctors who practiced chemical medicine instead of herbs, were the quacks. So it depends on your point of reference.

So, I humored my friends and professors, lying to them if necessary and doing whatever it took so I could continue to do this program - my life depended on it. I did not feel guilty about it. These were crucial times. So, I hid everything. In fact, I learned to be creative, keeping supplements in the pockets of my white doctor's coat and popping them when no one was looking. I thought it ironic that I kept such supplements in my doctor's coat - things considered quackery by the medical profession, but which were keeping me alive. I slipped into stairwells since nobody used them.

I would duck quickly into bathrooms and take my supplements. Just for kicks, I popped those supplements right behind the doctor's backs as we were making morning rounds. I was getting reacquainted with thrill-seeking and it was fun. I mused at how no one ever turned around when walking from room to room. The doctors were so absorbed in their complex doctor talk that they hardly noticed anything else around them. I always made sure to be the last person in the group so no one was behind me to see this. That wasn't hard to manage - it was hard enough to walk as fast as everyone else, although I was gaining strength.

My friends knew I had a hard time walking up stairs; in fact, they would make jokes about it, and so would I. I knew that if I freaked out my friends out too much, they wouldn't want to be around me anymore.

CHAPTER 9

The Beginning of Life

Controlling the Uncontrollable

So, I started my first rotation at the beginning of life: birth. Obstetrics was the most physically demanding rotation of medical school, since those babies all chose to be born at night or very early in the morning. So, we were scheduled to be in the hospital all night long to deliver the babies. This was after we had already been at the hospital since 7 that morning. After we had stayed up all night delivering babies, we were expected to drive downtown to the free clinic and see gynecology patients.

I don't know why in my sick, sleep-deprived condition that I didn't wreck my car and get killed. During these scheduled times, about once every five days, I worked around 33 hours in a row. There was no designated sleeping area for the students, and we heard that it was considered a "bad attitude" to sleep even if there were no babies to deliver, so none of the medical students slept.

Since we were at the county hospital, most of the patients spoke Spanish, and we had to pick up as much medical Spanish as quickly as possible. There had been no course on Medical Spanish during the first two years of school. There were no translators, and there were few Spanish-speaking nurses or technicians who had time to help. Most of the time, I found myself using a lot of hand motions, and shutting the little phrase book because it didn't apply. I was not qualified to interview patients in Spanish, and I was not supervised. For the most part, we were on our own to learn these things.

When the ladies came in to deliver, they automatically went to Triage. Triage is a big room where decisions are made as to where specifically a woman should go to deliver her baby. Some would go to surgery to have an emergency C-section, some would go to the regular delivery room, and some would go to intermediate rooms where they would receive more attention than in the regular rooms. In the triage area, there was a nurse's station around which were many chairs. The students and I used to sit around the large counter and discuss theoretical patients as well as what to do with the current ones. We also heard stories about other students, and what had happened to them on this rotation the night before.

We learned that our attitude was very important, and that we should not complain about anything or make waves. Attitude, we were told, made up a large part of our grade. Grades were very important because they would determine which residency program we would be accepted to after graduation. If you wanted your top choices, you had to have good grades. We all knew that a bad residency could be a horrible nightmare. So, we learned that in order to make a good grade, we had to do <u>more</u> than what was required of us. We should always be asking constantly to stay and see more and do more procedures. We should always be reading a book on obstetrics and gynecology and be asking questions about it. The recommendations were that specific.

The only problem with this was that it was impossible even for my friends to be that industrious for so many hours in a row. After a while, the words would start to move around on the page, and you didn't know what you were reading anymore. Now, I realize, that we were being brainwashed with all of the sleep deprivation, the talks about "attitude" and not complaining or making waves, and being worked harder than our ability to perform. We were to memorize minute details even if they didn't make sense, and we were to believe everything we were taught.

No one ever questioned the minute details, even though they would seem to contradict other information that we had learned last week. No one had time to think about it or question it. The sleep deprivation made it easier to accept things as fact even when they seemed not to make sense. Things were just accepted. After all, we were learning the most scientifically advanced, effective form of medicine that existed. We were told we were the brightest, smartest, best students in the country and that we were hand-picked to come to this medical school. Who wouldn't have wanted to believe that? We were ego-tripping.

Everyone would begin to get cranky and irritable around 3:00am and I was downright hungry. To take time off to eat was not encouraged, and when I did so, I was made to feel that that was highly unusual. I began to feel like a robot. I was supposed to be doing the same thing the same way as everybody else. So, it was like this code of silence; if you wanted to get a good grade, and everyone did, you shut your mouth, and worked yourself to death. If you got hungry, you raided the vending machine, but you certainly didn't take any time to sit down and chew your food. We learned to always look like we were studying.

The residents and the professors would ask us questions about anatomy or the progression of labor, a rare birth defect, or some other obscure fact and we were always expected to know the answers. They called it "pimping." No one liked to get "pimped," but everyone did, even in the middle of the night after a hard day's work. Even in the middle of the morning after a hard day's and a hard night's work. Yet, even with this treatment, the professors were careful to mention that at this university, we were being treated particularly well, and that this pimping was really nothing to be concerned about. Just enough to confuse a sleep-deprived brain. The logical connection was that we were lucky to be going to this medical school where we were treated so well compared to the other schools. Just more brainwashing. Pimping is designed to intimidate students and make them feel bad about what they don't know. It puts students in a catch-22 position and makes them study even harder. The harder they push and study, the less they learn, and the more likely they are to accept the information as fact even if it doesn't make sense.

Each morning, there was conference to report on the previous night's activities, and a discussion of some topic that related to one of the cases, like what are the signs and symptoms of preeclampsia? I always dreaded these conferences because I was no longer able to think after having stayed up all night. I couldn't remember where the conference was, or when it was, and resorted to following my friends. I had no idea what was being said at those conferences, and my dread was that I would be called on to recite the complications of anencephaly (a condition in which a fetus develops without a brain.)

My eyes would begin to shut and I would shake myself out of it. *This is important - I have to stay awake* I told myself. But, it was impossible. I knew the answers, but was too tired to understand the questions. Later on, my friends would tell me they saw me sleeping. I didn't know, but I found out later that I wasn't the only one. I don't know why it is part of the training to push people beyond their physical limits. I don't know why this is acceptable. It seems we are killing off our medical doctors faster than the rest of the population by putting them through this experience where they learn to push themselves this hard, and after years of doing it, their bodies give out and they have a heart attack or a stroke.

I'm told the average age of death for a doctor is 55 to 58. For the rest of the population it is 79 for men and 81 for women. Doctors have no idea how to care for their bodies in order to live, but yet somehow the entire population relies on them to give out health advice. What is the old adage - "Do as I say and not as I do?"

Some amazing events happened on this rotation. One was that I saw ultrasounds being performed that showed the tiny image of a baby. I could see the tiny arms and legs, and we always questioned whether the protrusion was a penis or part of the umbilical cord. This would be a very important fact to relay to the parents. Life is such a miracle. I knew it without a question when I delivered my first baby. The baby was over 10 pounds, and I literally had to brace myself to be able to pull it out. When he came out, he was so warm and slippery and miraculous that I almost dropped him. There was this live thing squirming in my hands. I realized then what a precious gift it was to be alive!

Sometimes, though, I would see the miraculous process gone awry as I would see ultrasound pictures of fetuses with birth defects. Now, I understand why the birth defects happen. The mother was eating the standard American diet and was exposed to chemicals and medications that cause birth defects. There are so many birth-defect-causing chemicals out there in the environment that it would be pointless to name them all - they're everywhere. They are part of the American way of life. I know that a fetus requires a tremendous amount of nutrients and energy, and lacking these, will develop as best it can under the circumstances with defects, or it will abort itself.

I had the opportunity to observe a few Cesarean sections, one of which was combined with a tubal ligation (commonly called "getting your tubes tied"). I remember watching the doctors pulling the baby out of the uterus, and out of the abdomen. They sliced the lady's abdomen wide open to get the baby out. I remember how bizarre it looked and how violent the cutting was. After the baby was born, the doctors began to dissect around the ovaries to tie the tubes. Mainly, medical students just observe surgeries, answering questions about the anatomy they are seeing and about the disease or procedure they are watching. They have the honor of holding the surgical wound open (called retracting the wound) while the surgeons work in there. So, the students don't really do any surgery.

The doctors asked me if I wanted to tie off the tubes as if that was a privilege. I obeyed as ordered. As a medical student, it is again considered a bad attitude to refuse to do something you're asked to do. I was later told that medical students are commonly asked to tie the tubes, because if the mother encounters any problems due to the procedure, it's not the doctor who actually ends up getting sued. It's the medical student. It's the individual who actually tied the tubes. A technicality, I assume. The medical student is at the lowest end of the totem pole.

We learned that babies delivered by C-section have more problems with their lungs, and with pneumonia because they don't have their lungs compressed by going through the birth canal during a regular vaginal delivery. Because their lungs didn't get compressed, the mucous was not squeezed out of them, and this would cause a potentially life-threatening pneumonia. Since it was a major surgery, there was also the risk of the mother dying, hemorrhaging, and having severe infections.

I also learned that the C-section rate was a lot higher than I had expected. I thought this was some sort of emergency procedure for when the baby or Mom's life was at stake, but they happened all the time for what I considered to be no good reason. According to figures from the National Center for Health Statistics, in 1988, C-section deliveries rose to an all-time high of 24.7% of nearly 4 million live births. For midwives and home births, the C-section rate is only about 3%. It is a difference in techniques used to birth a baby that make such a difference.

In Dr. Robert Mendelsohn's book Male Practice (now out of print), he describes the danger of having a woman deliver a baby while she is lying on her back. This position compromises the blood supply to the baby. This causes fetal distress which shows up on the fetal monitors. Because of this, the doctors put a special monitor on the scalp of the fetus to monitor it more closely. But, to get this monitor on the scalp, the doctor has to break the fetal membranes and cut into the baby's scalp to attach it. This understandably causes more distress. Because of fetal distress, the doctors decide they will have to do an emergency C-section. After the surgery, they claim they have saved the lives of the baby and the mother. They just put the mother in the wrong positioning for giving birth. The proper position for giving birth is squatting. There are even special birthing chairs for this purpose. Natural healers have known this since the beginning of time.

I saw natural healing improve people's physical and emotional health, whereas I saw the modern medical system destroy doctors due to competition, sleep deprivation and to many responsibilities.

There are people on this rotation I will not forget. Dr. Roughie, a first year intern, worked with us on our obstetrics rotation. Before her medical training, she had previously been a nurse, and she was quick to point out that she had gone to one of the most prestigious medical schools in the state. She seemed to have an inferiority complex about having been a nurse, as nurses are somewhat looked down on by doctors. In medicine, there is a rigid hierarchy, and in this hierarchy, people feel they must fight to keep their place.

Sleep deprivation can bring out the dark side of people and I began to see hers. On the outside, she seemed to be a rather pleasant person. In fact, she was rather pleasant-looking. Interns, though, are usually more sleep-deprived than 3rd year medical students, and I know that it can be extremely difficult to hold yourself together under those circumstances.

One morning around 5:00 am, I was sitting around the nurses' station. All of the babies had been delivered. There were no patients in triage, and no work to be done. I could not look at my obstetrics book any longer, and I could no longer think straight. Drowsiness overcame me, and I thought maybe I'd just lean on the counter with my arm propping up my chin. Somehow I drifted off into a nice warm nap.

Suddenly, I was jolted awake by a hard slap on my back, and Dr. Roughie was screaming at me, what did I think I was doing falling asleep in triage where people could see me? People might be shocked to find out how badly the medical students are being treated! No point telling her there was no designated area for students to sleep; I was so tired, I couldn't even remember this fact. With her finger pointing accusingly at me, she bellowed, "If Dr. Sloth had caught you, he'd have been a lot harder on you!" Everyone knew that you didn't want to make Dr. Sloth angry.

Dr. Sloth was a short, very overweight man whose area of expertise was gestational diabetes (a temporary diabetes that can occur during pregnancy). I had begun to wonder if this was his specialty because he was trying to find a magic pill to cure diabetes in pregnant ladies so he could cure his own. I suspected he was diabetic because he was very much overweight, and it's hard to be that overweight without being diabetic.

I tried to pull myself back to consciousness enough to apologize so that it would blow over. It's a tradition to abuse the medical students. It's an initiation. The mentality is if you're going to be a doctor making life and death decisions, you're going to have to be strong enough to do it, and the way we toughen you up for this job is by abusing you.

So, Dr. Roughie was on a roll, not realizing she was just acting out what was going on implicitly in all of the doctor's minds. The next morning, we would do rounds, and then we would drag ourselves to the other side of the hospital to do rounds on the ladies who had recently given birth. For delivering babies the night before, we wore the basic hospital scrubs. We would forget to don our doctors' coats for rounds until Dr. Roughie would yell out at us, "Go back and get your doctor's coats right now! You're doctors now! Act like it!" God forbid we would look like nurses. Dr. Roughie was a real doctor now; she wore her doctor's coat with pride, and everybody was going to know about how important doctors are, because she's a doctor and not a lowly nurse anymore. So, we went back and got our coats to humor her. A nice lesson to demonstrate the hierarchy. We were egotistical medical doctors in the making.

A sink or swim attitude pervaded our training. When we were told to do something, before we could open our mouths to say, "I don't know how to do that," the resident had to run off to catch up on his own patients with which he was horribly overloaded. There was not enough time to explain to us exactly what we were doing. We had to figure it out on our own. But we knew we weren't supposed to upset the patients, the doctors, the attendings or the residents. It was a pretty tall order keeping everyone's wishes straight.

After trying so hard to please everyone and spending the whole night and the next morning delivering babies and making rounds on the ladies postpartum in the hospital, I would walk out to my car to drive over to the Cody White clinic. Many times I would marvel at my ability to stand up after such a night, as I half expected to pass out on the way. I was so numb and so removed from my body that I was barely there. As I was taking steps, I was amazed at my ability to do so. Somehow I always arrived at the clinic and back home again.

I really don't remember much about gynecology clinic because most every time I went there when I was very sleep-deprived. We were to conduct patient interviews at the clinic and perform basic gynecological exams. My morale was low and I didn't want to see patients due to being so exhausted. I began to relate to derogatory stories about patients, identifying with stories about how someone's patient was hysterical and there really wasn't anything wrong with him. I lost my feeling for patients because all I could think about was food and sleep. Feeling cranky and irritable like everyone else, I tried not to show it. After all, it's accepted that this is the training.

One day, an attending told us to look under this microscope to see what a trichomonas looks like (a microscopic parasite that causes vaginal infections). In my sleep-deprived confusion, I felt like slamming his head into that microscope because I was so angry. I had not been allowed to sleep and I was being required to function this way. But, we did all of the examinations, again with minimal instruction due to lack of time. I noticed that the recommended diet for ladies with gestational diabetes was full of meat, dairy products and other highly processed foods. These were the kinds of foods which contribute to gestational diabetes in the first place. This was merely a low carbohydrate version of the same standard

American diet that makes us all sick. I made no comments about how I thought this medical treatment for diabetes, pregnancy and everything else was ineffective. I smiled, and indeed all of us smiled and did our jobs without too much of a fuss.

Although I was able to avoid the topic of my personal healing program up to now by shutting my mouth, there came a time when I was forced to discuss it.

Dr. Chestnut was one of the attending physicians who supervised the residents and medical students. He seemed to take an interest in me right away because of the hue of my skin. My skin had turned bright yellow from the large amount of carrot juice I drank daily -- a harmless condition known as hypercarotenemia. The skin, and especially the palms of the hands and the soles of the feet, turns yellow.

Jaundice, caused by liver inflammation or infection, also causes the skin to turn yellow, but the difference is that the whites of the eyes also turn yellow, whereas in hypercarotenemia, the whites of the eyes stay white. I had been this yellow for a while, and other people had begun to notice. In fact, people on the street and in the hospital would stop me and ask me why I was so yellow. It was hard to keep repeating myself that it was just a harmless reaction caused by the carrot juice.

Actually, it was a detoxification reaction. The carrot juice stimulates the liver to release old poisons and chemicals, as well as old bile pigments which are yellow. The liver releases the yellow pigment, which goes into the bloodstream and works its way out through the skin, causing the characteristic discoloration. Claire had told me that the more yellow a person turned from the carrot juice, the sicker and more full of toxins they were. Many people at Claire's clinic turned yellow; it was expected and considered a normal part of doing the Program. Claire said she had put hundreds of people, maybe thousands, on this amount of carrot juice, and they always turned yellow if they were very toxic, but after their body was cleansed, they didn't have the yellow coloration anymore, even if they drank the same amount of carrot juice every day. She also told me I was the second yellowest patient she ever had.

Dr. Chestnut asked me why I was so yellow. Well, the answer wasn't easy. I mentioned that I had been very ill until I found a nutritionist whose care I was under, who told me to drink carrot juice, and that it was working, and I was feeling much better. He had to have selective hearing, because the moment he heard sick and natural healing, he put them both together and made the connection that the carrot juice was what had made me sick in the first place. I tried to correct his mistake, but he was on a rampage. *Those natural healers are out there hurting people* is what I'm sure he was thinking, and was the common medical attitude towards it. He was a very pushy man, and tried to intimidate me. It worked. I know he had the thought that he was going to save me, so I give him credit for that.

He was very tall with striking white hair, a deep, reso-nating voice that almost shook the room when he spoke, and he wore eyeglasses for farsightedness that magnified his eyes to about twice their size. He looked and sounded like a man with which you did not want to disagree. Dr. Chestnut thought that I had hepatitis and he insisted that I go upstairs to the lab to get tested because he did not want me to infect the other students or the patients. I tried to tell him that it was hypercarotenemia and that I didn't have the yellowing of the whites of my eyes. He didn't much care for my argument, and he couldn't care less about the whites of my eyes.

He was a man on a mission: to save this medical stu-dent from the dangerous clutches of fraudulent quackery. I was ridiculed in front of my peers. To refuse his intrusive questions and comments would have been considered having a poor attitude, and grounds for administering a bad grade. After all, how could I not take responsibility for having some-thing infectious that could spread to my patients and to my fellow students? He insisted that I stop drinking the carrot juice at once.

I very dutifully carried out his orders *except for the carrot juice part.* I smiled and nodded, and as I was preparing to leave the room to go to the lab, I heard him say, "Yes, I need to check my own lab values, too, because my last cholesterol count was 300 and my triglycerides were 500." These were grossly abnormal lab values showing his ill health which was due principally to his poor diet. I knew that if he started drinking carrot juice and stopped eating so much cholesterol, he wouldn't have this physical condition. That made me rather indignant that he had the gall to give me dietary advice when his own health habits were actually killing him. I knew mine were healing me.

I went upstairs to the lab to be tested for hepatitis and the next day, the results showed I did not have hepatitis. I tried to tell him before, but he had not been willing to listen. One thing I did learn, was that as soon as I would say the words "natural," "vitamins," or "healing foods" to a medical doctor, he would automatically stop listening and try to get me to stop doing whatever natural, nonsensical, unscientific, unproven quackery that I was doing.

I went home that evening, got out the carrots, turned on the juicer, and I decided to make extra ounces of carrot juice every day to drink just for him. There has never been a single person hurt by carrot juice, only healed. He could not quote one single research study to me about how I was harming myself with carrot juice because they do not exist.

Then, I had a problem. What was I going to do the next time I saw this doctor? My rotation brought me in contact with him at least a couple of times per week, and the rotation was 6 weeks long. I decided to be sly and not to make waves. This is the typical medical student way. When I saw him walking down the hall, I turned around and walked the other way. I ducked into empty patient rooms, I struck up conversations with the people standing around, and I avoided eye contact. I did anything I could to avoid another interaction with him. I was fairly successful at this until the last week of the rotation.

At that time, I was still very yellow, and I was drinking even more carrot juice than when we had first spoken about it. He caught up to me one day, grabbed my arm and pulled me aside. Expressing the full gravity of the situation with the seriousness of his tone, he interrogated me, "Have you stopped drinking the carrot juice?" Petrified at his size and seriousness, I was able to mutter a sheepish "yes," a full nod, and a convincing smile. He replied, "Good, because you look a lot better!"

I told Claire and the other patients this story and they all laughed. They say what you don't know won't hurt you, but I'm sorry to say, that what he didn't know about me DID hurt him. If he would've questioned me, and started doing some natural healing methods on himself, he would be healthier today. He would not have high cholesterol or triglycerides, and he wouldn't be taking any medications. This is an easy thing to heal -- naturally. But, doing nothing about it will lead to deadly heart attacks and strokes, as well as other diseases in the body.

Of course Claire had another story. She told me about the only person yellower than me, a technician who worked in a hospital setting. Her superiors kept forcing her to get tested for hepatitis and it was always negative. Doctors have no understanding of what carrot juice actually does in the body, and can't seem to remember their own teachings about the obvious differences between the physical signs of hypercarotenemia and the physical signs of hepatitis. Maybe it's because they're too sleep-deprived when they learn it to actually remember it.

Doctors do on occasion save lives. There was a lady who came into the emergency room in labor. She was a cocaine addict, and her blood pressure was so high from the drug that it threatened her baby. Her placenta begin to peel off of her uterus prematurely and she began bleeding profusely. The fetus was over 15 weeks early. But, once the placenta starts coming off, the baby has to come out because the placenta is what feeds and sustains the fetus. They delivered the baby by emergency C-section. As the baby came out, the doctors placed it in the clear glass cubicle. The baby was dark purple and was no larger than the hand of the doctor trying to listen to its heartbeat. There was a huddle of doctors and nurses around the baby and a flurry of activity. They were all trying valiantly to save its life. It was a striking example of how babies turn out when the mother abuses her body with drugs.

But recreational drugs are not the only way to abuse a body. Everyday, Americans consume large amounts of re-fined sugar, salt and flour, meat, artificial colors and flavors, household chemicals, coffee, tea, alcohol, cigarettes, medica-tions, and soft drinks. The baby could've been premature for any of these reasons, but this lady just so happened to be ad-dicted to cocaine. There was a heroic effort to save the baby, but I heard later that it died. It was just too early for it to be born. At least they were able to save the mother. She could have bled to death.

As the pregnant ladies came into the hospital, the other students and I would screen them, looking up informa-tion to see if they had gotten good prenatal care. Good prena-tal care consisted of prenatal vitamins, ultrasounds, and any vaccinations if needed. We were upset if the mothers didn't receive any prenatal care, concluding that they were being irre-sponsible.

Regardless, the Hispanic ladies who came to deliver their babies in the county hospital, those who didn't drink heavily or do any drugs, seemed to have the easiest births with the fewest complications. What was amusing to me is that two times during this rotation, ladies came in after having given birth at home. They didn't come to the hospital sooner because they had no idea they were pregnant. They were teen-agers, and no one had ever taken the time to explain the facts of life to them. When they went into labor, they felt as though they were having strong menstrual cramps or maybe even the stomach flu, but then out came the big surprise, which was when they called the hospital. The point is that they had no prenatal care, and yet they delivered healthy babies.

During obstetrics training, doctors learn how to push themselves beyond their physcial limits. Many doctors tell me now after they've experienced some sort of illness due to the incredible amount of stress they've placed on their bodies from the lack of sleep and working long hard hours, that they didn't realize what they were doing to their bodies. They didn't know they couldn't handle that much stress. Since everyone during their training works those hours, it just becomes accepted. As a result, they usually develop some sort of chronic illness, or have heart attacks and strokes. Seeing 50 patients a day is somewhat stressful. Remember, the average age of death in doctors is 55 which is much younger than the rest of the poplulation.

According to the April 15, 1998 issue of JAMA, a survey of 1,277 second-year-residents listed in the AMA's medical research and information database revealed that ten percent of residents indicated sleep deprivation was an almost daily occurrence. They averaged 56.9 hours a week on-call at the hospital, and 25% of residents said they were on-call more than 80 hours a week. Seventy percent of residents reported observing a colleague working in an impaired condition for which lack of sleep was the leading cause (56.9%).

The American Medical Student Association publishes a magazine called The New Physician. An article, entitled *Doc Grumpy*, related that long hours and fatigue may not harm patients, but it may harm physician outlook, states Dr. Michael Green in a report in the Annals of Internal Medicine (Vol. 123, No. 7).

In 1984, 18-year-old Libby Zion died under the care of sleep-deprived residents at New York Hospital. A series of residency reforms resulted, but residents are still working long hours. Green, who studied the reforms, concluded that the main consequence of grueling residencies was poor physician attitudes but *not* poor clinical performance. "The primary consequence of prolonged hours seems to be that overtired house staff develop undesirable and unprofessional attitudes," he writes. "Reform should focus on changing the institutional ethos that promotes cynicism and dislike of patients."

I wonder if the experts can recall volumes of memorized material after having stayed up all night and still keep a professional attitude. The atmosphere of cynicism and dislike of patients exists, so isn't it logical to assume that the dislike of those patients would affect the care that they get? Sleep deprivation is a specific technique used worldwide for brainwashing. It is very effective for that. It could be considered a form of violence or even torture. If you tell people they are not allowed to sleep, wouldn't you consider that to be a form of torture? How should we expect the residents to react?

The scientists have already proven that lack of REM sleep, the part of sleep that includes dreaming, eventually results in insanity. Over the short term, this lack of REM sleep results in irritability, short tempers, poor concentration and many other problems. Doctors' "dislike for patients" doesn't randomly appear out of nowhere! Why don't we ever look to the obvious for what's causing the problem - lack of sleep, abuse and mistreatment.

During the gynecology part of the rotation, I learned all of the different birth control pills, doses of estrogen, and progesterone. I also learned that there was a particular, extremely common drug given to women for menopause that comes from pregnant mare's urine. I thought about how disgusting that is, especially considering that menopause is not a disease, and it's not an estrogen deficiency. I also knew that there were herbs that ease this transition, not only relieving the symptoms, but balancing the body's entire hormonal system, not just the sex hormones, without side effects such as CANCER from estrogen. Wild yam, chaste tree berry, blessed thistle, dong quai, black cohosh, and many other herbs help nourish and balance a woman's reproductive organs.

The young girls were guinea pigs for a new drug that came out that provided birth control for a few months at a time. It was implanted underneath the skin of their upper, inner arms. There really wasn't much research done on it and after a while, it became apparent that there were a few side effects that had not been mentioned during the supposed clinical trials, like heavy menstrual bleeding and headaches. Eventually, some gynecologists refused to prescribe it anymore. It made me wonder, after taking this drug and screwing up their hormonal cycle, did these women have problems conceiving afterwards?

That led me to the fertility clinic. Many women were infertile because their thyroid was either underactive or overactive. Easy enough to fix -- just give synthetic thyroid hormone to those whose thyroids were underactive and radioactively destroy the thyroid of those whose thyroids were overactive, and then give them the same synthetic thyroid hormone.

The interesting thing about thyroid medication was that every time I saw a patient who was taking it no matter what rotation I was on, they always complained to me of symptoms that they weren't getting a big enough dose - dry skin and hair, fatigue, gaining weight, depression, lethargy, etc. The inability to lose weight greatly bothered them. They told me their doctor checked their blood and told them their thyroid was fine, and that their dose was perfect. I always wondered it if was just that the medication didn't work well, or if the laboratories were messing up the blood tests. Naturally-derived thyroid medication used to be used with better results, but no longer was used presumably because the marketing people for the synthetic version had more money and more push. That doesn't matter to me now; I wouldn't even suggest the supposed natural version because it's not necessary when people change their lifestyle and detoxify their body.

People with overactive thyroids had had their thyroids "nuked," but were amazed that even though the doctors said that this would essentially "kill" their thyroid, part of it grew back and was STILL overfunctioning. After all of that radioactivity, after all of that poison - could we wonder why they were still sick? Most of the time, this "nuking" would destroy too much thyroid so that not enough hormone was being produced, and then these patients would have the same problem with their medication as the ones with the underactive thyroid.

Later, I learned about an herbal formula that helped infertile women conceive in around one to two months' time. Also, they didn't give birth to multiple babies at one time, putting their lives in danger, like the modern fertility drugs do.

I know that if women did some thorough bowel cleansing, their large intestine wouldn't become so enlarged with back-up bowel movements, squashing down on their uterus and ovaries and causing so many female complaints like menstrual problems, irregular periods, infertility, vaginal infections, endometriosis, etc. I saw so many support group meetings for people to discuss how their female problems were incurable and how they had tried the latest drugs and surgical procedures, only to still have their problem.

Psychiatry

Take Your Drugs and Stop Manipulating Me

I learned very interesting psychiatric theories while I went through my psychiatric rotation. I learned about how "the psychiatrist is always right and the patient is always wrong because they are not mentally competent." This gave the psychiatrists I knew free reign to do or recommend whatever therapy they wanted and to use a sort of emotional blackmail to get their patients to do as they said because of course the psychiatrist knew what was best for them and was of course trying to help them. Nowhere during my medical school experience and the numerous rotations I went through, did I see a patient so willing to give up any personal resistance to a medical treatment as I saw here. Patients did whatever the psychiatrist said to do, with the only exception being the teenagers (they wouldn't do what anyone said -- not their parents, their doctors, and not even their friends). Many of the psychiatrists I met were sour and cynical individuals who tended to blame their patients for being mentally ill, as if they thought their patients could just "snap out of it" if they weren't so "ornery."

Psychiatry is an very elusive science. The mind cannot be dissected. It argues; it contradicts itself, and it changes its mind. What we call "normal thinking processes" are merely what we believe everyone around us exhibits. We call abnormal whatever is out of the ordinary. But, is this fair or right?

Do we really have life so figured out that if someone

comes to us with a paranormal experience, we can rightly call him a lunatic? How do we know that that person has not tapped into another dimension of life of which we have no direct knowledge? How do we not know that there may be people out there more sensitive to energetic vibrations in the environment who can read minds or talk to the dead? How can we be so arrogant to assume that the life we live, (the one where we get up every morning at the same time, kiss our spouse and go to work, go home, drink beers, hang out with our friends or family, play sports, engage in a hobby, watch TV, go to sleep) is everything there is to our existence and that there are no other meanings or interpretations about life that differ from the prevailing opinion?

How do we tell people that if they don't think and act the way everyone else does that they have some sort of mental disorder? What we do in psychiatry is tell people that there is something wrong with them, which in this society carries a sort of stigma to it, thereby reinforcing a patient's sense of inferiority. Then, on top of it, we have the audacity to tell people that they have a "chemical imbalance," as if their bodies are so faulty that they very capriciously just decided to stop working properly, and as if it had no idea how to balance itself out.

We play with a very delicate system of neurochemicals, not knowing what the long-term effect will be from our interference with the body's own processes. Our patients end up dependent on our drugs for years the same way they can't walk on their own after having walked with the aid of crutches for so long. Their legs are withered and bony from disuse. Our patients' brains are withered and soggy from relying on psychotropic medications, medications that act specifically on the mind. One problem with psychotropic medications is that if one goes thoroughly through a Physicians' Desk Reference, one will find a whole host of extremely undesirably side effects, including the conditions they are intended to treat. For example, many antipsychotic medications can cause psychosis, and many antidepressants can cause more depression, and can aggravate mania in a person who has manic-depression.

If you introduce a neurochemical into a person's body, several things will occur. One is that the body will say, "Look here, it looks like I have enough or even an oversupply of this neurochemical, so I won't have to make anymore. Then, as long as that chemical keeps coming in, the body says, "You know, I still have enough, so I don't need to make anything." Pretty soon, the structures in your brain start to shrink (the medical term would be to atrophy) because if you don't use a structure, this automatically happens. You know that if you have built up your muscles by going to the gym, and then you stop going to the gym for several months, that your muscles will begin to shrink from disuse.

I know several people who have been on antidepressants for years - they've even switched over to the newer, supposedly more effective ones, and still they are not able to get off of them. However, they've never tried a natural approach. They've never tried to revive their worn-out, toxic, malnourished brain cells with the proper nutrition and a detoxification program. I know anything is possible with natural healing and a strong enough will to execute it.

Psychiatrists and doctors in general have a tendency to blame patients for being ill. It gives them a sense of security. It makes them feel as if they have control over a disease. One of a doctor's worst fears is dealing with a terminal disease and psychiatric disorders. There is nothing the doctor can do or say, no treatment he can give that will alter the course of the disease. A doctor is trained to have mastery over human bodies - he can go in and take out parts, put in new parts, put in medication that will stop wheezing in just a few minutes, sew back together a body that's been severely traumatized in an accident, yet has absolutely no control over a terminal disease, and most psychiatric disorders. A doctor tends to take this personally and this fact makes him subconsciously feel like a failure. But, if it's the patient's fault he's sick, then it relieves that burden off of the doctor to save the patient. "That cynical and outspoken patient has sabotaged himself with his or her living habits and therefore nothing I can do will save him, but that doesn't have anything to do with my competence as a doctor." Then, a doctor doesn't have to lose faith in medicine because it's not working, since it's the patient's fault for "somatizing".

Somatizing means to be have multiple changing symptoms, yet there is no physical problem that explains the symptoms, meaning that there is nothing physically wrong with the patient that the doctors can find with their tests. I say these things and yet, I've caught myself doing exactly the same thing, saying silently to myself that it's the patient's fault for not healing because I've given them every treatment available out there. Well, we've given them every toxic drug out there for their condition; am I really surprised that they weren't healed?

My psychiatric attending physician had a very critical attitude. She used to barrage me with criticisms about the lunch I brought from home. She was also very overweight. When I first came onto the rotation, she told me there had been another medical student who had rotated through this department who believed in vitamins and health food, and that she thought it was a load of crap. I think she even used those words, coarse in her manner as well as with her words. She rather growled at me, "You're not one of those health food *freaks*, are you?" I pushed back her verbal assault with a quick, yet timid "no" and changed the subject to a current psychiatric patient on the ward. She thought she could win by intimidation. Maybe she thought she was saving me from the fraudulent quackery, too.

I developed an intense dislike for this attending physician, as I began to see her sense of ethics through her actions. There was a young lady in her 20's who had had a kidney transplant who came into the hospital for severe depression and psychosis – in other words, she was hallucinating.

She saw wedding rings when she hallucinated, and it was sad because I think it was her way of grieving because she did not think she was good enough to marry due to her physical condition. Steroids also cause a lot of changes in a person's physical appearance. You get acne, you grow a mustache if you're a woman, your muscles shrink and get weak, you have emotional highs and lows, you get osteoporosis, and you're always fighting infections because your immune system is depressed. You gain a lot of weight and retain water easily. The doctors put her on a tricyclic antidepressant which caused her to have urinary retention (she couldn't urinate). This is one of the common side effects of tricyclics. Of course, she also got dry mouth and constipation, too, which worsened her condition. Urinary retention for too long can back up into the kidneys and cause kidney failure, and she only had one kidney. She had been on immunosupressive drugs, including steroids, ever since her kidney transplant when she was two. Since steroids can cause psychosis, I felt it was a pretty clear-cut case of steroid psychosis.

The attending wasn't interested in how medical drugs cause psychiatric conditions; she wanted to use *more* drugs to fix it. She decided on lithium. I vehemently disagreed with lithium, as one of its side effects was kidney damage, and this lady was already severely compromised with her kidney function seeing as how it was the transplanted one. *I thought this system of medicine was supposed to be scientific.* This patient's treatment was flying directly in the face of common sense because of "supposed" science. The attending felt it wouldn't hurt her, and figured she could just monitor the patient's blood tests to check her kidney function to see if any damage occurred. The problem with that is that by the time you see evidence of damage in the blood test, the damage has already occurred!

This attending was one of those who blamed her patients for being mentally ill, and she made several comments to that effect. I wish I could've made a formal complaint, but that would've been making waves. That young patient will be on medication for her kidneys, and for psychosis, for the rest of her life. The causes of her illness were never considered, and so she got a chemical cocktail instead. Even more medication was piled on top of the old ones that were making her even sicker while seemingly controlling her symptoms. After a week or so, she was discharged from the hospital, branded with the label of mental illness that was really created by the medical profession. Natural healing might have saved her kidney in the first place at the age of 2, and none of this would have happened. I know of many who have been able to take themselves off the transplant list because they healed themselves naturally.

There was another lady who came into the hospital with manic depression. She had taken several kinds of antidepressants over the past twenty years of her illness. The only reason she was admitted here was because she told her home health aide, "What's the use of trying anymore?" Immediately, she was considered suicidal and was given the choice - either check yourself in voluntarily to the hospital, or we will commit you involuntarily. Sometimes, I think we would just rather drug our elderly patients so they don't complain, rather than listen to their valid concerns. Of course, she had been ill with manic depression because the real cause of her illness had never been addressed. She was merely given drugs to cover up the symptoms as much as possible. Control and cover up symptoms are what doctors do best with their drugs.

The attending decided that the indicated treatment for this lady was ECT (ECT stands for Electroconvulsive therapy). This therapy consists of attaching electrodes to the head, which send electric currents into the brain which cause the person to have a seizure. The patient is secured to a table with leather straps and medicated heavily so that they will not have the involuntary spasms that cause them to thrash about and hurt themselves. The main complaint after having a series of these shock treatments is loss of memory. I knew exactly how that felt! How irrational it is that we think we can heal people by giving them seizures! As I watched the procedure being done, I felt as if I were living in the Dark Ages. Her body twitched slightly because she was not medicated heavily enough. When she awoke after the ECT, she began to complain of a sore throat. She felt so horrible that she did not want to have any more therapy.

The attending was too clever for that. Remember, the psychiatrist is always the right one, and the patient is the wrong one because they're considered mentally incompetent. She figured the patient was trying to manipulate her by feigning illness. The attending assured her and cajoled her into doing more therapy, smooth-talkking her by telling her how much this therapy was going to help her. So far, it just seemed to be making her much more irritable and even sicker. Reluctantly, the patient agreed, and we were all back down in the treatment room watching her have seizures all over again. Again, she complained of a worse sore throat. The attending still thought she was complaining just so that she could get out of more ECT. She made more remarks about how the patient was very manipulative.

Eventually the patient won out. She steadfastly refused to have any more seizures. Thank goodness. Seizures cause brain damage! She was released from the hospital, but not before she complained of a cough in addition to the sore throat. Again, the attending said something about how the patient had no reason to complain and was being manipulative. She prescribed some sort of cough suppressant to make the "supposed cough" go away, saying she was only prescribing it to make the patient happy, and she really did not think this lady was ill at all - just complaining too much.

Two days after her release from the hospital, we received a call that the same patient was being readmitted to the hospital because of pneumonia. The lady must have taken the cough medicine because suppressing a cough can lead to pneumonia. Her body was trying to get rid of toxic material in her lungs, but the doctor forced it back in with the cough suppressant and made it worse. The patient gave signs and symptoms of being ill all along, but since she was a mentally ill case, no one listened to her. Even I couldn't make the attending listen.

Ironically, during this rotation, there was very loud construction work going on near the psychiatric wing that went on all day long. All of that noise was a stress to the patients, and every single one of them complained about it. Was anything done for these people? Their nervous systems were already on the edge, and now there was this unbearable noise of drilling and hammering all day long starting in the early morning. I feel certain that most of them would have been better off at home than at this loud hospital. How is a person supposed to take this noise and get well from their psychiatric condition at the same time? The noise was *really* bothering *me*. In Europe, when they want to help someone with a psychiatric condition, they put them in a quiet, peaceful place.

There was a very nice, quiet, and reserved lady in her 40's who was admitted to the psychiatric ward for paranoid schizophrenia. She had delusions that her neighbors were trying to kill her by putting boric acid all over her apartment, and that they were sending X-ray beams through the walls at her, and other things. The interesting thing about this patient was that one day, I came into the hospital and found out that her blood sugar had gone down into the 40's (normal is around 100).

The doctors, in their ignorance of what might have caused that, were just going to fix the number. If her blood sugar was low, they would just give her more sugar. She was given the traditional chocolate, vanilla and strawberry-flavored "nutritional" canned shake and told that it was good for her because it had vitamins in it. Also, it contained refined sugar and processed dairy products - just full of poison. Great, now she's going to have to take sugar every few hours for the rest of her life.

When the blood sugar hits that low, as many diabetics can tell you when they accidentally take too much insulin, people begin to get confused; they can even pass out. The brain cannot run on any other fuel than glucose (a sugar). Since this particular lady did not pass out, that told me that this had been a chronic condition that had been going on for some time. No wonder she couldn't think straight. No wonder she was having delusions. She had not been getting enough glucose to her brain. Traditional medicine does not recognize hypoglycemia as a bona fide medical condition.

They were giving her sugar-filled shakes which were just causing an outpouring of insulin from her pancreas which would cause the blood sugar level to go low all over again. Did they really think they were helping her? No one considered that her liver was very toxic and her adrenals were very weak, and that she could have done some liver cleansing to relieve her hypoglycemic condition. There is a strong link between the functioning of the liver and the functioning of the brain. When people do natural liver flushes, they consistently notice improvements in their clarity of thought, their memory, their depression, anxiety, etc. If everyone knew how to do liver flushes and colon cleansing, psychiatric conditions would be extremely rare, and I believe the psychiatric profession would run out of cases.

But, they wanted to stress out her liver even more by giving her antipsychotic drugs. Antipsychotic drugs commonly damage the liver. If the liver functioned perfectly in the first place, people would not become psychotic. A psychotic person already has compromised liver function, and the doctors pour more chemicals into the body that have to be processed by an already sick liver which over the long term, makes the condition worse.

I remember how all of the psychiatric drugs were so highly toxic. I would consider them to be the most toxic drugs in the medical profession besides chemotherapy for cancer. In the pharmaceutical industry's efforts to make better drugs that didn't have so many side effects, I remember they had just come out with a new drug for psychosis. It caused major drooling. People who took this drug walked around with saliva dripping out of their mouths. There will never be a synthetic drug made that does not cause side effects, the reason being that they are synthetic. Our bodies are designed to accommodate natural substances, and when it encounters a synthetic chemical, it tries to get rid of it as quickly as possible. There are symptoms that occur during this process of poisoning and the body trying to get rid of the poison, and these are called side effects.

The Endocrinologist

Since Claire had told me I was in adrenal failure, I thought finally there was some physical condition that the doctors could document. The medical term for adrenal failure is Addison's disease, or adrenal insufficiency. I searched out an endocrinologist and told her that there were hours out of the day that I was unconscious and couldn't be accounted for. She asked me if I had ever had any evidence of having seizures. I didn't know what it was like to have a seizure. I really didn't know anything about them, so I said no. She continued to administer the test used to determine if I had adrenal insufficiency.

After the test was over, she wanted to have me take a steroid pill to see what my reaction was to it. She wanted to see if it would make my blood pressure go up. If I responded in a certain way to this steroid pill, it would help her make the diagnosis. I was dead set against taking any pharmaceutical drugs anymore, so I told her I couldn't take that pill. Later, after putting in several calls to her to try to find out the results, all I got was a brief response that it was negative and she never returned any of my other calls. I assumed she had considered me a non-compliant patient, a patient who is troublesome and doesn't do what the doctor tells him to do. I had asked Claire if I should have taken the steroid pill for a few days to help the diagnosis, and she screamed at me, "No!"

She had already seen the results of people when they took those steroid pills. My body had already seen the results of taking steroid shots in the past. The doctors try to tell their patients that if they keep taking the steroids for something like 14 days or less, then they don't get any effect on their adrenal glands, and therefore, a short course of steroids is absolutely harmless. They are only poisoning you for 14 days instead of 15. These numbers are quite arbitrary. What is the point to how many days they put some synthetic chemical in your body? They're putting it in - period.

But something the endocrinologist said stuck in my mind, and the next time I saw Claire I asked her, "Is it remotely possible that I could be having these seizures? I mean...I know I'm not really that sick, and I couldn't be having them without knowing it, right?" She answered, "There's one way to find out," and she told me to begin taking a choline and inositol supplement because it would begin healing my nervous system.

I took the supplement. Two nights later, I had fallen asleep on the floor again, and I awoke at midnight with an unbelievably intense pain at the base of my spine. I figured I must have bumped myself in my sleep again. The pain did not abate. It continued and it worsened, then spread all the way through my spine. As it traveled upwards, the air was being squeezed out of my lungs at the same time as I heard myself saying on my forced exhalation, "No..." Then, my arms flew up in the air and over my head and my entire body just started shaking very rhythmically for about 2 minutes until everything stopped.

I had no idea what had happened except that it was the most horrible, excruciating pain. Afterwards, my shoulders were really hurting. I had hyperextended them during this seizure, but not enough to dislocate them this time. I thought I was in a hospital bed, and that there would be a nurse coming by any minute to check on me. But, no nurse came by. I realized that I was very confused, but I did not want to move. I looked at the clock and saw that it was around midnight. Mostly, I did not want to believe that anything had happened.

The next day, I went in to see the family doctor again to tell him what had happened. He called it a borderline seizure. I really don't think there's anything called borderline seizures. You either have them or you don't. He suggested a CAT scan of the brain and an electroencephalogram (EEG) to determine the cause of the seizures. Finally, someone took me seriously. But, now I didn't believe in medicine anymore, so I declined the tests. I just wanted to know if it really was a seizure. I already knew that no matter what it was, brain tumor or not, that I would have it taken care of it with natural methods only.

I don't know what possessed me to go back to the hospital psychiatry unit to work that day. It was crazy. But the truth was that I had been going to clinics every day, even with the seizures, the only difference being that now I knew I was having them. I walked into the elevator in the hospital and was greeted by a resident I had worked with in the past. He asked me how I was, and I didn't see any reason to mince words, so I just told him, "I feel pretty awful; I just had a seizure this morning."

Granted, that's not the most common response to the question, but he didn't believe me. He said I probably thought I had a seizure but likely I was just feeling shaky from drinking too much coffee. Too much coffee??? I didn't drink coffee, and I knew I really did have a seizure the night before. One prevailing attitude that some doctors have about medical students is that they dramatize their problems and make it so that they believe they have a serious disease when they really don't. True, a few medical students get convinced that they have the disease they just studied, but this is not common.

When I went to see Claire, I told her of my experience, and she said that it was a seizure. She also said that a person taking the supplements would be healed of the seizures by first becoming aware that they are happening. This is exactly what happened. From then on, I began to wake up right at the end of a seizure, knowing what it was. Now I understood the bruises and the dislocated shoulders came from the seizures in the middle of the night, in the afternoon, and after school. I understood exactly the effects the seizures had on my body, and especially on my mood. I understood exactly how my arms moved during a seizure so that my shoulder dislocated itself. I paid attention to the messages my body was sending me. I listened. The entire two-year struggle of trying to figure out what was wrong was falling into place. I was beginning to understand.

At the end of this rotation, my group decided to celebrate by going to a Mexican restaurant for happy hour. I was feeling stronger and wanted to just pretend that I could be social. I came along and ordered water, knowing that I'd be the only person there not drinking alcohol. Actually, no one noticed.

This is when I met Marco. He had gorgeous dark, wavy hair, a perfect nose, warm, hazel eyes, and a muscular, fit body. He was an accountant who was friends with some of my friends. He was so beautiful that I didn't think he would ever give me the time of day. We were sitting at the opposite ends of a very long table. While we sneaked glances at each other, I bemoaned the fact that he must already have a girlfriend.

After a few hours, my friends decided to go to a party. As everyone was getting up and saying their good-bye's, I was briefly introduced to him, we shook hands and parted. I heard that he had gone to another house with his friends. While I was at this party, one of my friends received a call from someone at the other house who said that this guy really wanted to know more about me. He eventually came over that night, and we got the chance to chat. My friend told me I didn't want to go out with him because she just found out he was divorced and had two kids. It didn't matter. I thought he was the best thing since sliced bread.

As we were leaving the party, he asked if I wanted to get a bite to eat. It was 2:00 in the morning, and I told him I was kind of tired. He told me that was okay, and the sweet way he said it made me change my mind, and since that point, I was like putty in his hands.

The only place open was a 24-hour taco restaurant. The only thing I could eat was a plain bean burrito. He asked me, "Is that the only thing you want?" and I was trying not to tell him all the gorey details about why I couldn't eat red meat or processed food anymore.

I don't know how in the worst time of my life, the best man in my life came along to keep me company and give me lots of love and support, but it happened. The whole sordid story eventually came out, but he didn't run away. He wasn't scared at all. He said he didn't care if I went to a natural healer as long as it was helping me. For some reason, he saw me as more than just a tangled mess of symptoms. He told me to do just go ahead and do whatever it was that I needed to do. I never got so much unconditional love in my whole life.

I remember Claire telling me that my body couldn't handle chicken, much less red meat. There was way too much sodium in chicken. At that point, I didn't know what else to eat but fish. Our first date was at a seafood restaurant. Whenever Marco and I would go out to eat, it became a standing joke that he would ask me where I wanted to go, and I'd say, "Where can we get fish?"

When he asked me out on our first date, I told him I couldn't go because I had to go to school that day. He seemed rather puzzled that I couldn't go, but he said okay. I went to school that day, and no one was there. No one was there because it was Sunday. I was still having so many problems thinking that I didn't even know what day it was.

Ophthamology

Watch as They Slowly Go Blind

Throughout the rest of my third year rotations, I slowly discovered the reasons which led to my decision not to practice medicine. I saw what medicine did to people and I simply couldn't do that.

My ophthalmology rotation was at the Cody White clinic that was the clinic for lower income people. They charged very minimally and on a sliding scale. I remember the depressing air of the clinic, and the defeatist attitude of the patients. They didn't have the money to have a good life, so why even try?

It seemed like everyone went through the mill with the same thing. There were so many diabetics, and they all got the laser surgery to burn the back of their retinas to stop hemorrhaging. The retina lines the back of the eyeball and is crucial for eyesight. They were called flame hemorrhages because they looked like tiny flames when you looked at the retina through the ophthalmoscope. The blood would damage the retina in a tiny spot, causing a blind spot. · But, the surgery itself would cause blind spots, as well.

The diabetics would come in regularly to have this surgery done repetitively, each time, losing a little more of their vision. They were slowly going blind because of the hemorrhages, as well as from the surgery. The surgeon cauterized and stopped the bleeding and left a scar on the retina. The scar caused a blind spot. No one ever told the patients they had the chance to completely heal their diabetes, and that they didn't have to suffer from these complications.

As I examined eyes, I began to notice the irises of their eyes. The chiropractor whose books I had read had perpetuated a system of iridology which originated from a medical doctor in Germany. With iridology, one could tell the condition of each organ in the body. I began to observe and correspond people's health conditions with the markings in their irises, confirming for myself the validity of iridology. Its accuracy surprised me.

I observed a few surgeries during ophthalmology. There were several cataract removals, another type of surgery that could have been avoided with natural healing. There was a one-year-old baby who had a rare tumor of the eye called retinoblastoma. Even with removing the entire eyeball, there was no guarantee that they would get the entire malignant tumor. I often wondered why they hadn't gone to a natural doctor down in Mexico, since they were Mexicans. If the mother and her husband had taken Mexican herbs and detoxified their bodies before conception, she wouldn't have had a child with such a serious tumor. That child was fated to die. During the surgery, they didn't get all of the tumor. The doctors said that it had spread too much.

In an attempt to stop a further spread of the cancer, the child would have radiation to that area of his face. Because of this, one side of his face was not going to grow, and if he survived, he would grow up with serious deformities of the head, looking like a mutant.

We learned about a particular drug used for rheumatoid arthritis and the side effect was that it caused retinitis pigmentosa, normally a genetic disease. Luckily, the disease stopped when they discontinued the drug. I saw not just one, but a few of these patients on this drug. Because this side effect was so serious, every time a doctor prescribed this drug, the patient was sent to ophthalmology every six months to check for signs of this horrible disease.

The topic of my research report during this rotation

was retinitis pigmentosa. Later on, I learned of a great American herbalist, who designed an herbal formula back in the 1950's or so. It was designed to be used as an eyewash several times a day. Using this eyewash, people had had their cataracts fall off, their glaucoma go away, and their nearsightedness and farsightedness improve or totally disappear. His herbal formulae were so effective that they gave a baby sight who was born without optic nerves. Using this herbal eyewash, that baby grew optic nerves with which to see. The herbalist died in the 80's, leaving behind many students, many of whom still recommend the use of this formula.

Urology

Surgery, Blood and Burning Prostates

The next four blocks were surgery rotations; these would be difficult, since the hours were atrocious. Surgeons have a reputation for being domineering, arrogant and insensitive. Not everyone was that way, but most were. Many felt that in order to be highly skilled at cutting someone open and playing around in there, you had to be pretty full of yourself to think you could do that. You don't think it's disturbing to cut open live human beings? I remember all of us had nightmares after taking gross anatomy our first year. It was very disturbing. But, we learned to cover up and suppress our real feelings about the cutting. We made fun of the bodies, and somehow that distracted us from thinking of that person as a valuable human being that we could potentially kill with surgery. There is always that risk of death during a surgery. If the patient is a fat, overweight slob, we don't have to worry if we think we're not up to the task of doing the surgery perfectly.

I heard so many insults thrown at patients while they were under anesthesia, or just that sort of talk amongst surgeons while the patient wasn't around to defend himself. I suppose this sort of talk, under the circumstances of surgery, would be better than the surgeon breaking down into tears and crying, "I can't do it; I can't control all the variables; what if something goes wrong?" At least that would be truthful.

The most shocking thing I saw in medical school was surgery. I had no idea it was so careless. The way the sur-

geons put things back so sloppily, it didn't seem very respect-
ful to the patients. Nor did I expect the horrible smell of
burning flesh to be so bad.

The doctors used an electrocautery unit that cauterized
any bleeding capillaries or blood vessels when the wound
would start to bleed. I asked one of the nurses if the people
being operated on knew about the electrocautery. It was so
bad that comments were made about it during surgery. I figured this was a major part of the surgery, so the patients must
have been informed about it, but the nurse replied that the patients had no idea.

It felt weird that the patients didn't know all of the
trauma involved in performing a surgery. First, the skin is cut,
then the flesh is charred as it's bleeding, then something is removed. There is all of this cutting and destroying tissue to get
to the needed area. Sometimes, the surgeon took out pieces
of tissue or fat that he thought the patient didn't need, said
something to that effect, and moved on. Next, especially at a
teaching hospital, the patient is sewn up by a resident who had
barely learned how to do it. There was so much trauma to the
tissues as the needle and surgical thread repeatedly pierced
through the flesh. I often marveled at how people survived all
of it.

On top of that, the surgeons didn't mind at all what
they said about the patient during the surgery. Some surgeons
were nicer about that than others - some were outright dispar-
aging. Surgery is so unnatural that many made jokes about the
patient to protect their sanity. If not, they would think about
the person too much as actually being a human, and that they
were actually entrusted with the life of this human being while
they were operating. How far out of balance have we gotten
that cutting into each other with knives is considered normal
and routine?

There were remarks made about the weight of the patient, "Oh and he doesn't need this extra bit of fat," the surgeon would say while removing it -- "Every little bit helps."
Sometimes they were referred to as whales. Being morbidly

obese was a contraindication for surgery. It was too risky to do the surgery on someone in such poor health. But, for the less obese, that didn't stop the constant criticisms. The surgeons would joke around, expecting us to laugh along with them. This made me very uncomfortable. Smile and go on. I could hardly smile, let alone go on.

I always thought it was extremely disrespectful, and I knew that I had read in numerous places and was even taught during my basic sciences years, that some people can remember what is said in the operating room during surgery and can be affected by it.

After surgery, it is so common to have a fever that they taught us the most common causes and we memorized them for tests. Most of them started with the letter W - Wonder drugs (the pharmaceutical drugs prescribed by the doctors), Water - urinary tract infection, Wind - atelectasis (failure of part of the lung to expand), Wound - wound infection (we even learned the most common types of infections). There are so many complications that can happen as a result of surgery that it would be impossible to list them all and have the terms be understood by the lay person, but the following are some examples. Urinary retention (can't urinate), kidney failure, respiratory failure, bleeding, pneumonia, cardiac arrhythmias (heart beats irregularly), heart attack (causing many to die suddenly right on the operating table or within 24 hours of surgery), depression, dementia, delirium (disorientation and hallucinations), aspiration pneumonitis (inflammation of the lungs caused by accidentally inhaling backed up stomach acid during surgery), postoperative hernia (intestines protrude through the surgical opening even after closure), excessive scar tissue that obstructs the bowels (leaving some patients with mild to severe and possibly life-threatening constipation), blood transfusion reaction, a worsening of an already existing disease, at least 20 different types of infections, and the sutures could come undone causing many problems and sometimes requiring another surgery to correct it. It seemed like most of the time spent on surgery rotations was watching how slowly people recovered, and how long they had to stay in the hospital recovering. With the empty, nutritionless hospital food they were given, it was no wonder.

It didn't take me long to discover that a surgeon's training allows him to see the human body as made up solely of separate, unrelated parts. Due to this Leggo theory, as I called it, a surgeon can mix and match those pieces in many different ways. However, in natural healing, I learned that every organ affects the other, and that none of the parts should be taken out. The tonsils and appendix were very important parts of the immune system, the tonsils being the only organ in the body which can produce antibodies to the polio virus. I had learned all of this information in the first few years of medical school, but somehow, it all got conveniently forgotten come surgery time. The doctors taught me about how important the gallbladder is in digesting the fats in a meal, and if removed, a person would have a difficult time digesting fatty foods - for the rest of their life. Then we learned about how to take it out.

Doctors gave little importance to the immune system, and in many diseases, it was considered to be harmful. In some cancers, autoimmune diseases such as lupus, lung diseases, and others, medicines were actually given to suppress this "dangerous immune response." Yet, I remember learning specifically that the T cells of the immune system specifically killed not only viruses and fungi, but also cancer cells. Maybe everyone was too sleep-deprived to notice this obvious contradictions. I didn't understand why they were making such efforts to suppress the body's own healing powers. I knew that the successful natural herbal treatments, the ones that were successful, involved strengthening and boosting the immune system. I knew my friend Charlene who had lupus had healed so well because her immune system was getting stronger.

It was as if the medical school professors had taught it so rapidly that no one had time to sit down and think about all of the contradiction. Otherwise, the professors may also have learned it so rapidly that they never had time to actually think about it, either. They were repeating it exactly the way they had learned it.

When I rounded on many surgical patients, many times they would beg and plead to see their doctor. They'd tell me things like they hadn't seen their doctor in 4 days. The surgeons would check briefly on the patients so early in the morning that half of the patients were not awake yet. In fact, one of the residents told me just to make sure they were still breathing, and if so, then they were okay. For many of the ones who were awake, the surgeons would sometimes not even enter the room, but merely asked if they were okay, and that they had no time to talk now.

As surgery would start at the crack of dawn, I had to get up quite early in the morning. It was part of my job to check on the patients before they were brought in for the operation. The surgeries would usually always go past the scheduled time, resulting in an even greater level of exhaustion by the doctors and students at the end of the day. Surgeries routinely got postponed.

Surgeons notoriously work so many hours that there have actually been studies done - one of which revealed that some first year residents in New York were working hours well exceeding the limit of what's humanly possible, especially given such a high level of stress during those hours.
Source: American Medical News June 15/22, 1998

According to the study, "...examiners from the New York State Dept. of Health paid surprise visits to 12 teaching hospitals and found that more than a third of residents are working more than 85 hours per week. State regulations limit resident work hours to 80 per week, averaged over a four-week period.

The state's 80-hour work limit does not apply to surgical on-call time if hospitals provide documentation that on-call residents are receiving adequate rest. Yet the survey found this documentation was absent in hospitals. Many surgery residents were working more than 95 hours a week. Department investigators confirmed that surgical residents were not receiving adequate rest while on call.

Sixty per cent of surgical residents statewide were working more than 95 hours a week. In New York City hospitals, 77% of surgical residents worked more than 95 hours per week.

"The survey revealed widespread abuse of the resident work-hour limits, particularly among surgical residents in New York City."

"Are we surprised? Absolutely not." Darren Duvall, MD, chair of AMA Resident Physicians Section, was quoted as saying, "We have known this is going on and we're glad the state has documented it...Currently, a resident cannot say without fear of reprisal, 'I am too tired to work.'"

Joseph Valenti, MD, a resident at Buffalo General Hospital and a member of the RPS governing council said the results actually indicated that conditions in New York were *better than they had been in the past.*

I never saw so many surgical complications. Before every procedure or surgery , the patient signed a consent form saying that they understood the risks of the procedure/ surgery, and that they agreed to have it done. This was usually a rushed encounter which involved little more than saying that the risks were infection, pain, bleeding and a maybe a few others. No patient ever expected to have the complications that they had. The surgeons had seemed so confident. The surgeons said infection - they didn't say maybe your life could hang delicately in the balance while you sat in intensive care because of a massive infection while they tried five different types of antibiotics until they finally killed the infection causing the peritonitis. The surgeons never mentioned that the pain could be so severe that you would be begging for more pain medication, yet the residents were hesitant to give you too big of a dose. No one ever said, "Look, you can make some changes in your diet, take some cleansing herbs, get on an exercise routine, and do some water therapies and emotional healing, and you'll get well."

There was TURP after TURP after TURP. There were so many TURP's being performed, it was as if patients were just being run through the TURP mill. TURP, an acronym for transurethral resection of the prostate, is performed on men who have enlargement of the prostate gland. The prostate can enlarge so much that it begins to slow down and even obstructs the exit of urine from the bladder. The urine then backs up into the kidneys, and over the long-term leads to kidney failure, necessitating kidney dialysis for the rest of the man's life. Because the medical doctors didn't know what caused this enlargement, all they knew how to do was keep slicing off bits of prostate. Since the cause was never addressed, the urologists would tell us that every few years or so, the same patients would return to the hospital for yet another TURP, as their prostates had continued growing and enlarging during that time. The best they could hope for with medicine and surgery was to **control** this problem, but not to **heal** it. With natural healing, we can get to the cause and heal it.

During a TURP, the surgeon takes a long metal rod, and goes up the penis with it. Next, a cautery loop comes out of the rod, and the surgeon "shaves off" parts of the enlarged prostate. He is actually burning the flesh off. There is obviously the stench of burning flesh in the operating room during this procedure. One of the residents told me he actually enjoyed the smell of burning prostate. Lucky for him, for a surgeon working so many hours, at least he had a great attitude.

After this procedure, every man was urinating blood and sometimes chunks of tissue for at least a day up to about a week or so. All had a hollow tube called a Foley catheter inserted to drain the blood-filled urine immediately out into a bag. Because of the surgery and also because of the catheter, there was a risk for urinary infection. Antibiotics were very freely prescribed to prevent this.

There was a man who had prostate cancer who was admitted to the hospital to do a TURP, but he decided against it. He told us he was just going to eat pumpkin seeds because he had heard they were high in zinc and good for the prostate.

I thought, *he needs a lot more than pumpkin seeds if he is going to get well from this*, as cancer is a total breakdown of the body no matter what type it is. Maybe he didn't realize that all those years of eating meat and other animal products filled with hormones - natural and unnatural - were the real cause of his prostatic enlargement. Doctors know that certain hormones cause the prostate to grow.

He probably had not heard of cleansing his intestines as they totally surround and affect the prostate gland. He never read the latest research linking the consumption of red meat to prostate cancer. One of the treatments for prostate cancer is a hormone blocker and/or castration to remove the testicles which produce testosterone (the male sex hormone). I thought how silly it is to remove body parts and block the hormones. This is a bit drastic! Why don't they just stop putting growth hormones in their bodies! (They were getting these from meats and other animal products.) If they would stop putting the hormones in, they wouldn't have to block them. I always thought it strange that no one caught on that the growth hormones used to raise animals were being ingested by the public when they ate meat, causing serious effects. Growth hormones make things grow. This is why we call them **growth** hormones. Why wouldn't they make the prostate, the breasts, and tumors and cancers grow?

Most importantly, he would have done very well to take saw palmetto, an herb that is known for shrinking the prostate, diuretic herbs (herbs that make you urinate) as well as other herbs. In fact, the November 1998 issue of the Journal of the American Medical Association recently included a research study, showing that saw palmetto produces similar improvement as the prostate drugs in urinary tract symptoms and urinary flow and caused fewer adverse treatment reactions (Saw Palmetto Extracts for Treatment of Benign Prostatic Hyperplasia, JAMA; Vol 280, No. 18, pp. 1604-1609.). This is new news to medical doctors, but is old news to herbalists and other natural healers.

I saw one patient in the urology clinic who told me he

and his wife had started taking some sort of tree bark, getting rid of their diabetes. I told him, "Don't tell anybody what you told me, or else they'll tell you to stop taking it. And you just go right on taking it if it's helping you that much." I used to ask for *everything* the patients were taking, and they would tell me because I would really listen and not judge them. There were so many that had tried or were trying herbs and natural healing, and their primary doctors and their specialists had no idea because they had never asked.

I remember a man who had had a prostate removal for prostate cancer who was in the hospital for the entire 6 weeks of this rotation. The common complications of having the prostate removed are impotence and incontinence which can be seriously debilitating. When the surgeons did the surgery, they accidentally cut a part of his bowel with the scalpel, so when it healed, his bowel made an abnormal connection with his bladder. Every time he went to urinate, fecal matter came out instead of urine. He was so depressed. Since the surgery schedule at this particular hospital was booked months in advance, he had to wait a long time for the surgeons to do another surgery to correct it. He stayed in the hospital while he waited because it was free at this hospital.

The surgeons told him that maybe the fistula (this abnormal connection between his bowel and his bladder) would heal, and that they wanted to wait a few months to see if it did before they did another surgery. They didn't tell him the surgery schedule was so full. They didn't tell him that fistulas do **not** heal on their own without surgery. He became more depressed every day. He was so depressed that nobody wanted to go into his room anymore to check on him because he would just cry every day. They even sent a psychiatrist in there to talk to him because it was suspected he was suicidal. Talk to him about what? That he could possibly live with fecal matter coming out whenever he peed?

It wasn't until months later when I was on the intensive care rotation that I saw this man again. He was in intensive care because he had finally had the surgery to correct the fistula. But he ended up with a severe abdominal infection called peritonitis as a complication of the surgery. He lay there for several days, and his wife came in to visit him, crying over his seemingly lifeless body as he was attached to all sorts of tubing.

I continued my weekly visits as a patient to Claire's clinic and talking to more and more of her clients. Claire and I began to talk about different cases, and she would tell me stories about how a particular patient died because they wouldn't believe her that they could be healed naturally, so they tried to mix her routines with medicine. Something terrible usually happened. Sometimes the medical therapy is so toxic, it kills people no matter what herbs they take to compensate for it. The philosophies of natural healing and of medicine are so vastly different, it is very difficult to use them together. But people try. I've heard they were trying to get essential oils used during surgery for stress relief and to fight infection in the hospital. The oils may kill the infection, but the surgery may still kill the patient.

Cardiothoracic Surgery

Life On The Line

I woke up at 3 am in order to do my health program, as well as to get in early to the hospital to do rounds. To say I was exhausted would be putting it mildly. As I turned off the alarm, it was still pitch black outside, and I would apologize profusely to Marco for having woken him up with the alarm. He didn't complain a single time. I never understood how it was that he could be so understanding and so compassionate, but he always was. I would complain about having to get up over and over, and he would just let me lie there. After a couple of minutes, I would force myself up against the exhaustion, both of us amazed that I could get up this early and work.

The patients were the sickest on this rotation. Most of them had bypass surgeries because their coronary arteries were clogged with cholesterol. Not one single time did I ever hear a doctor tell one of these patients that maybe they could change their diet or eliminate cholesterol from their diets to heal themselves. After the surgery was over, I would visit the patients on rounds, and they would be sitting up in bed eating turkey and mashed potatoes, and I thought to myself, *Oh my God, this is why they're here in the first place!* The hospital's idea of a low fat, low cholesterol meal included - meat! Dairy products! Eggs! Since there were cholesterol-lowering medications available, no one cared about eliminating cholesterol from the diet. However, most of those drugs caused liver damage. In fact, the one cholesterol-lowering medication I learned that did not cause too many harmful side effects was niacin, a B vitamin that stimulated circulation. Its cost was ridiculously low, and maybe this is one of the reasons it was rarely prescribed.

Not only were the meals atrociously prepared, irradiated (scientists know that radiation causes cancer) and chemically laden with pesticides, chemicals, hormones and artificial and refined ingredients, but the patients would pick at them because the food tasted so horrible. For that reason, I guess they figured they'd never be able to eat a low-fat, low-cholesterol diet, so they never tried. I tried to stay at least five feet away from any hospital food. Maybe the cafeteria staff should have read some of the books in the health food store in order to prepare some foods that actually had some life in them instead of overcooking them, and if they started off with pure, unrefined ingredients, then the patients would recover much sooner. If the patients had followed that sort of diet in the first place, they may never had ended up there!

I know of many people who have reduced dangerously high cholesterol readings just by eliminating animal foods from their diet. The program outlined by Dean Ornish, MD is almost mainstream, and many insurance programs now cover it. This medical doctor discovered when he put his patients on an almost cholesterol-free diet that their cholesterol levels went down and their atherosclerosis reversed itself, sometimes even in severe cases. He combined this food program with some moderate exercise and meditation and relaxation every day, and was able to get great results. He says the cholesterol buildup in the coronary arteries is reversed 90% of the time. His program sounds exactly like what a naturopath would recommend.

Animal foods are the only foods that contain cholesterol. Most patients had no idea where cholesterol was, much less where it came from. Steak, chicken, turkey, sausages, seafood, fish, milk, cheese, eggs - these are all either animals, or came from animals. People just kept following the recipes of their parents, and ate what their parents taught them to eat. Nobody questioned that Americans eat probably more animal foods than any other country on the planet. We have one of the highest rates of disease in the world, too. There is certainly a link there. I saw most patients dying from their own ignorance of what it was they were supposed to eat. They thought they needed their "protein", and their toxin-laden protein always came combined with a high percentage of saturated fat and cholesterol. Even the medical profession now states that high protein diets are not without their high share of saturated fat and cholesterol. They call these diets unhealthy.

The bypass surgery (they're called CABG's for short - coronary artery bypass grafts) was a massive surgery. During this surgery, the surgeon would slice all the way down the center of the chest with a scalpel. He would then use an electric saw, and saw through the center of the breastbone. Bits of bone dust would fly everywhere. After that, he would try to pull and yank with another instrument until the chest was all the way open. It disturbed me to see how violent it all was. I could see the skin wrinkled and stretched all around the huge, gaping hole, and it didn't even look real to me. Meanwhile, a resident was working on slicing the leg sometimes all the way from the ankle up to the thigh to remove a vein to sew onto the heart.

The main blood vessels coming in and out of the heart were cut open that required much skill because such large arteries, when severed could cause a person to bleed to death in minutes. If a doctor dared tell me this was a safe and routine surgery, I would laugh in his face. The arteries were attached to tubing to which was attached the bypass machine that pumped blood to the body. The machine had to accomplish this, since the heart would have to be stopped in order for the surgeon to sew vessels onto it. It's called a bypass because the coronary arteries are blocked off with cholesterol and fat, and the only way doctors know how to treat this is by taking a vessel that's not blocked off (the vein in the leg) and sewing it onto the heart, bypassing the clogged arteries that usually supply blood to the heart.

The coronary arteries are the only arteries that supply blood to the heart, and if completely blocked up, a person would immediately have a heart attack. Unless unblocked, that person would die, because their heart would die from lack of oxygen. It was a risky surgery because it involved stopping the heart by pouring a solution of potassium in the pericardial sac that surrounded the heart. They also filled the pericardial sac with ice to cool it down to reduce damage to the heart from lack of oxygen. The risks were death from a heart attack during the surgery, a lack of oxygen to the brain leading to brain damage, a stroke if a piece of cholesterol broke off and went to the brain, bleeding to death because the stitches didn't hold, and many more complications including the main one after surgery - pneumonia.

The medical student's job during this was to hold the heart still so the surgeon could sew the vein onto the heart. Easier said than done. My hand was in the ice-filled pericardium, and it was so cold that my hand went numb. Meanwhile, I stood on the edge of the podium (because that's all the room there was) between the surgeon and the anesthesiologist. The anesthesiologist and I were separated by the drape that separated the patient's head from the rest of his body. I kept getting smashed between the two while trying not to fall off the podium. My hand was completely numb while the surgeon kept yelling at me to keep it still, and I couldn't even feel my hand to know if I was moving it or not.

Meanwhile I was perspiring because I was right underneath the main surgical light. I kept getting hit in the face by the surgeon's elbow which caused him to contaminate the surgical field, requiring him to put on a new sterile sleeve. It happened so often, sometimes he didn't even bother to get a new sleeve. So much for sterile surgery. It was so crowded, I barely had enough room to stand so I could keep my hand on the heart and see where I had my hand (well, I couldn't *feel* where it was.) I wondered how other medical students found this experience. I really began to despise this extremely uncomfortable experience and tried to avoid it when possible.

After the vessels were sewn on, the large blood vessels would have to be disconnected from the machine and sewn back together. Since these were huge arteries, a mistake sewing them up could be fatal. The surgeon would then put the chest back together. He used wire to sew the breastbone back together. After recovery, many patients suffered from complications due to this wiring coming loose or piercing some vital structure. The patients had this thick metal wiring wrapped around their breastbone for the rest of their lives. I tried to imagine what it would feel like to have this inside of my chest, and decided it was too gruesome to think about. I could see the characteristic wiring wrapped around the breastbone on so many X-rays. I was shocked at the number of these X-rays I saw. Open heart surgery must be common, I concluded.

After the surgery was over, the patients would go to the recovery room. They would stay intubated on a ventilator, and it was the resident's job to try to get them off of it in the next day or two. This was easier said than done. There were at least two large drains that drained any fluid that accumulated during the surgery to the outside. (Imagine a piece of tubing that goes from the inside of your body through to the outside through your broken skin with the tubing actually stitched to your skin - OUCH! The patients all found it painful.) All of the fluids had to be careful monitored - what went in and what went out. We were forever checking lab values. It was incredibly time-consuming, and this is one of the reasons why we came to the hospital so early. There was a huge amount of data we needed to present at morning rounds.

Pulling out the tubes was a disturbing thing to do. But the patients were always relieved to have each one removed. After the initial risky period of one or two days, the next thing to watch for was pneumonia. The entire chest cavity had been opened and exposed to the air and bacteria, viruses, and other microorganisms, leaving it vulnerable to infection. There is no such thing as a totally sterile surgery - there are always at least some germs in the air that fall into the wound as dust.

There were always at least a few patients in the hospital who had contracted pneumonia after the surgery. It was a common complication. I saw other patients who had had more than one bypass operation because they never changed what they were doing that gave them this disease in the first place. They had breastbones that wouldn't heal closed, and I could see and feel their breastbone wobbling back and forth as they breathed. The doctors called it an "Unstable sternum."

The worst thing about this surgery was that there was no real patient education afterwards. The only education the patients received was how to take their medications. When the surgery was over, the patients were all placed on aspirin or another stronger medication designed to thin their blood (that was thick because of the saturated fat and cholesterol they were eating every day). That particular strong medication was used in another industry: as rat poison. When rats ingested it, their blood was thinned too much and they bled to death. Indeed, this was also a side effect when humans took it. An overdose could cause potentially fatal bleeding into the lungs, into the intestinal cavity, into the brain and into other areas of the body, as well. There are many safe herbs that have a blood thinning effect, but **none** of them ever cause the blood to be thinned too much or cause any bleeding whatsoever, let alone, result in death.

These people had no idea that the foods they were eating caused their heart attack. I repeatedly counseled patients on this **very crucial** point: how to avoid getting another surgery 5-10 years on down the line. You don't just expect that the new arteries won't just clog up again. So many Americans have had this surgery two or three times in their lifetimes at a cost of around $45,000 for each surgery. What is the national debt again? The statistics show that up to 15% of our gross national product is spent on health care.

Many people think after bypass surgery, they have received "all new plumbing." What they don't realize is that almost every artery in the body is in the process of getting plugged up with cholesterol and saturated fat simultaneously. I saw so many patients come into the hospital with a long history of having the cholesterol scraped out of yet another blood vessel. They'd have it scraped out of the carotid arteries (the arteries that supply most of the blood to the brain), or they had an iliac bypass surgery to bypass the clogged arteries to their legs. They had the cholesterol scraped out from nearly everywhere so they had scars all over their bodies. Each time, the surgery had to be done or else they would have lost some vital function or organ like their leg, their toes, or their brain. They were still at risk for strokes, kidney failure (when the delicate, small arteries supplying blood to the kidneys gets blocked off), and even sudden blindness when the arteries that supply blood to the eyes get blocked off.

Since having several mini-strokes causes people to have Alzheimer's symptoms, many people think they have Alzheimer's disease instead of the poor circulation to the brain due to a lifetime of eating cholesterol and fat-filled foods. Patients would come in for an iliac bypass, and they'd already had their carotids scraped out, and a coronary bypass, and still had a whole host of circulation problems. The coronary bypass did not solve the circulation problems in the rest of their bodies.

If I were a man facing this sort of risky, invasive surgery with so many complications and the potential to affect me adversely for the rest of my life, I would become a vegetarian in a heartbeat (no pun intended).

There was a physician's assistant (called a PA for short) in training with us, and she was treated badly because the length of her training was not "considered" to be as good as the training offered in medical school. Because of the hierarchy, she was looked down on. I frequently heard comments during school about how doctors thought other medical practitioners didn't know anything because they had not had as many years of training as they had. I called it professional snobbery.

Meanwhile, at that time, I was still trying to heal myself full speed ahead - healing crises and all. There were nights Marco and I would spend together when suddenly a headache would come on and nothing would stop it. I would be totally disabled with the pain. Sometimes he would get so concerned about me, he'd ask, "Don't you think you should go to the emergency room?" I would shout out emphatically, "NO!!!" In the delirium of my pain, I could do nothing else but scream. I would shriek, "They're only going to give me drugs, and unless I get to the cause of it, it'll keep happening over and over again, and pretty soon I'll be a pain medicine addict!" Sometimes the pain would be so bad, I'd worry if maybe I had had a cranial bleeding episode. I remember the professors talking about how patients describe their subarachnoid hemorrhage as the worst pain they had ever had in their life. That's certainly what it felt like. There I was crawling again and clutching at my head, wanting to rip it off. I would have pulled out all of my hair if I thought if would have helped the pain.

I hated to have him see me crawl because I was still having some of those days where after coming home from working in the hospital, I was so weak or in such pain that I couldn't stand up. Sometimes, I just refused to let him see me. I was a lot sicker than I ever let him see. I didn't want **anyone** to see me that way. I didn't want my family to know; I didn't want my friends to know; I didn't want anyone to know. I lived alone and I stayed alone except for going to the hospital and to the nutritionist's office, and being with Marco.

Other times, Marco and I would go for walks because I was trying to get some exercise. We would walk along the river when we'd approach some stairs, and I'd try to go up them, but my legs wouldn't carry me. At those times, I'd feel so frustrated and defeated, but Marco didn't say anything, he just carried me. He carried me whenever I got too tired to walk from the shortest to the farthest distances. Once when we left a theme park, he carried me all the way through that huge parking lot to the car. He kept saying that it didn't matter, and that he loved me anyway.

CHAPTER 14

Just A Routine Surgery
With Complications

There are some remedies worse than the disease - Publius Syrus, 50 B.C.

During and after Thanksgiving, I was on my general surgery rotation. The number of gallbladder removal surgeries during this time was phenomenal. The residents told me there was a surge in this type of surgery around the holidays, because people ate so much fatty, cholesterol-filled food. It was a surgery of overindulgence. I used to think it was a horrible shame that people should lose their gallbladders when there was a perfectly simple liver flush drink that they could make in their blender with olive oil, citrus juice and other foods and herbs that flush the stones right out. It amazed me that no doctor had ever heard of such a simple technique, since it would have saved millions of gallbladders. Liver flushes saved my own mother's gallbladder from surgery later on, and she, to this day, still has it.

Many surgeons lived up to their reputation of having bad tempers and being control freaks. I heard the words "Keep the horizon!" shouted at me in anger and frustration so often during the new laparoscopic technique to remove gallbladders. "Why can't you just get this? What is so hard about it?" Instead of making a long incision across the abdomen, four small holes were made in the abdomen through which various scopes, cameras and instruments were inserted, enabling the surgeon to see what was going on inside the patient's abdomen during the surgery. He normally could see well

when the abdomen was sliced wide open, but during laparoscopic surgery, there were only these small holes. Long rod-
like instruments were pushed into the holes with miniature
video cameras on the tips, and it was the medical student's job
to hold the video camera so that the surgeon could see what
he was doing in there.

One of the surgeons told me this laparoscopic technique was very difficult to learn and to perform, but a patient's
recovery time was quicker because it was less invasive. He
also told me that it is more likely the surgeon will make a mistake during laparoscopic surgery because it is so difficult to see
what they're doing through four small holes - even with the
miniature video cameras. He said that was one of the reasons
why many surgeons did not want to learn the new technique.

The only problem was that the camera showed everything upside down and reversed. Every time my arm moved
one way, the view would change the opposite way I expected
it to. The surgeon wanted me to keep the camera on a particular line of the liver that he called the horizon, and with all
of the movement of the surgery, it was just impossible! There
was nothing out of the ordinary about a surgeon yelling at the
staff during surgery. Medical students usually got the worst of
it since they were the lowest part of the totem pole. I heard
that this particular surgeon had graduated from the best medical school in the state, so he acted quite full of himself due to
this fact.

I really didn't appreciate being treated like a child, and
I was really fuming about it to another student when I realized
that he was standing right behind me. I don't know what or
how much he heard, but he never seemed to like me much.
Complaining like that about a resident would be considered
having a bad attitude which affect grades. Many medical students just swallowed their complaints about abusive treatment
because they were afraid of making waves.

According to the Sept.2, 1998 report of MS/JAMA
(Vol. 280, pp. 851-853), a survey of 1001 graduating medical
students at eight U.S. medical schools showed that a high

number of students had experienced harassment and discrimination during their training. Forty-six per cent of the students reported experiencing some form of harassment and 41% some form of discrimination from instructors or supervisors while attending medical school. Forty-one per cent reported nonsexual verbal harassment, while 10% reported sexual verbal harassment. Gender discrimination was reported by 29% of students, while 12% reported discrimination based on race.

According to the current American Medical Association President, medical schools have focused their curricula on technology and have abandoned their duty to instill young physicians with the principles of medical ethics (Only Return to Ethics Can Save Medicine, AMA President Says; *Internal Medicine News*, Oct. 1, 1998. p. 41). At another AMA annual meeting, the AMA president and panelists described medical learning as being "Long on science and technique at the expense of ethics and etiquette." It was mentioned in the AMA news that academic role models exhibited behavior such as belittling patients, berating underlings, undermining colleagues, and deceiving supervisors. A student panelist recalled one lecturer who complained for 30 minutes about his difficult patients (*Educators: Be Careful Not To Treat Students Unprofessionally*, American Medical News, July 6, 1998, p. 9,11).

I felt abused even more due to the way the doctors handled the next surgical patient.

A 14 year old boy was admitted to unblock his bowels and to figure out why he had severe constipation. In rounds with the chief of surgery, we discussed the possibilities. I suggested that it could be Hirschsprung's disease, which is a condition where a person is born with only a partial nerve supply to the colon - in other words, there are some nerves missing which are responsible for the movement of the colon. The portion of the colon missing the nerves does not move, and fecal matter backs up behind that point. I had the chance to feel this young man's abdomen and it felt like a huge hard rock. He must have been in a lot of pain. He could not have a bowel movement on his own for months at a time unless he had an enema. The surgeon thought Hirschsprung's disease was a plausible diagnosis, and suggested that we obtain a "tissue diagnosis," which meant a biopsy of his colon done so that it could be analyzed under the microscope to see if nerves were present or not. Some technician went up his colon with an instrument, and I'm sure it was painful, and forcibly pinched and cut off a piece of tissue for the biopsy.

While we were waiting for the results over the next few days, he received a "rocket booster" consisting of mineral oil and other medicines to unblock his colon. It did what the name said. The next thing we knew, he was in horrible pain, since the fecal matter was so hard that it cut him on the way out. He was only 14; I erroneously used to think only elderly people had constipation.

If he had Hirschsprung's disease, then the surgeons would remove that part of the affected bowel and reconnect the remaining edges. He would have had a colostomy temporarily which involves allowing a portion of the bowel to heal by diverting the fecal contents to the outside of the body and into a bag that would be glued on. I used to see a lot of patients with colostomies in the general surgery clinic. It was the worst clinic I ever worked in because I was dealing with everybody who had lost or was getting ready to lose parts of their body. I felt in the midst of mutants, as if it weren't real. I could smell those patients hundreds of feet away because inevitably, the bags would leak.

I thought colostomies and colon surgery were horrible things to do to a child, so perhaps he was lucky because the next thing I knew, the biopsy came back negative - there were nerves everywhere there were supposed to be. I presented this case to the chief resident of surgery, and told him the biopsy was negative. The surgeon took one look at me, said "Well, if it's not Hirschsprung's disease, it's psychogenic; send him to a psychiatrist!" Then immediately, "What's the next case?" Psychogenic means that the cause for his constipation was all in his head. I thought it was the rudest, most careless diagnosis I had ever heard. Just because he was no longer a surgical case, that meant he was a psychiatric case?

Since the child's mother told me he had been constipated since he was a newborn, I thought it strange that a person could have a psychiatric problem since birth. I thought it very strange indeed, and I knew the surgeon just didn't know the cause. Since a psychiatric reason was the catchall diagnosis for when a doctor didn't know the reason for something, that was the diagnosis he decided in on 2 seconds. He was a busy surgeon always in a rush. I wonder if he had any idea how much impact his 2-second diagnosis had on that child. It was one of those few times when I actually intervened. I was almost yelling at the child when I said, "Don't you ever let anyone tell you that this is caused by something being wrong with you mentally! I know a natural practitioner who knows how to help you." There were simple herbal formulas that stimulated the bowels to move regularly no matter what the cause.

I saw other children with colostomies and other diseases of the colon. There was a 16-year-old girl who was admitted to the hospital because of Crohn's disease. This was only one of many times she had been here. During one of those previous times, the surgeons had taken out portions of her intestines and given her a colostomy bag, and she suffered. She was having a dangerous bout with diarrhea - people can have it so severely and even bleed from their colons - that they can die. I still remember the surgeon screaming at her because she was sucking on a piece of candy. She was supposed to stop eating to allow her intestines time to heal, but she was so hungry that she couldn't stand it. She burst into tears, and cried that she just couldn't do it, and the pain was unbearable. "It's only one piece of candy," she begged. I just could not believe that such a young lady had been so butchered with surgery.

I found out that this condition, too, could be healed with herbs. This made it all the more painful for me as I knew if she had known about the natural way, she might have chosen it, and she would've kept all of her intestines intact. I knew slippery elm had healed many of colitis even hundreds of years ago.

I was allowed to observe other surgical procedures. One of those was a cystoscopy, involving the insertion of a scope through the urethra into the bladder to observe what is in the bladder. Sometimes it was ordered to determine why a patient was peeing blood. The causes could be anything from a bladder tumor to interstitial cystitis - a chronic inflammation of the bladder - to bladder stones to just a bad bladder infection.

Hearing loud screams, I gingerly opened the door to the procedure room. A woman who looked about in her 40's was complaining that she had never had so much terrible pain in her life, and how much longer was this going to take? She shrieked, "Oh God, oh God!" repeatedly. She said, "I don't know what I did to deserve this; I've never done anything that horrible - no kinky sex or anything!" The intensity of her screams frightened me. I assumed she had been given sedation but evidently it wasn't working. She was lying there on the table, and the surgeon had this scope up her urethra and was looking around with it. To have anything up your urethra is very painful to say the least, but she was lying on the table spread eagle, and I was embarrassed just to have her be so exposed to anyone who happened to open the door. So much for modesty. Sadly, she could have done some herbal kidney cleansing and cleaned out her entire urinary tract, and it wouldn't have mattered where exactly in the urinary tract the problem was.

At the end of each rotation, we would get a grade. It would be based on clinical performance, sometimes a written test and/or research paper, and of course, our **attitude**. I always received the highest marks possible on attitude since I had mastered kissing up. Not one of the things I'm proudest of, but definitely a necessity for a medical student. We even made jokes about it. In fact, we had a word for it. A student who is always doing more than he's supposed to for a grade, picking up extra responsibilities and studying way more than necessary we called a "gunner." I knew "gunners" during the first two years of lectures, but they never affected me. I would know one in Internal Medicine who would make my life a living hell.

There was a whole range of very diverse people in medical school, and our medical school was known for taking more unconventional applicants. The women made up 40% of our class. We also had older students, and people who had already had other careers. In our class, we had dentists, nurses, physical therapists, a cardiopulmonary perfusionist, an engineer, and other business professionals in our class, and we were proud of our diversity. We also had cheaters. It seemed our class was always taking the brunt for what the class ahead of us had done. We heard multiple stories about cheating at the other medical schools in the state. There was so much pressure put on medical students to make top grades to get into the residencies they wanted, that they cheated to get good grades.

Pediatrics

Suffering From Medical Misinformation

On to pediatrics where I began with Intermediate Care, a hospital unit which provided care somewhere between standard and Intensive Care. We saw many premature babies. There were so many of them in the incubators. We saw drug babies who were withdrawing from the drugs the mothers had taken right up to their birth. Then there were the complications - birth defects, pneumonia and other infections which started in the womb or soon after birth.

Before we could enter the intermediate care unit, we were required to put on gowns and scrub. Scrubbing meant washing your hands for a few minutes in a chemical disinfectant soap which came in a sterile package. There were foot pumps on the faucets, so we didn't have to touch the knobs to turn the water off. I thought that was nice that we killed the germs, but now when we touch the babies, we're leaving harmful chemical residues on their skin, making them sicker. The particular soap we used had been previously used to wash the babies, and it was found to be too toxic for them, since it was absorbed through the skin. *And I'm putting this on **my** hands everyday?!*

As we were rounding one day, the residents told us some history on the care of premature babies, including the use of incubators which contained high levels of oxygen. It was thought that this high level of oxygen would benefit the babies because they had such immature lungs that they had difficulty breathing in enough oxygen. It was an experiment.

Eventually, it damaged their retinas, and they went blind. It was not as simple as giving more oxygen to babies who couldn't get enough. I would have given the babies lots of herbs, love, touching, and most of all - MOM!

It was the medical students' job to evaluate all of the babies to see if they were normal. We checked their tiny heartbeats, their feeding patterns, their fontanelles - everything. The silver nitrate drops were so caustic that they caused a chemical irritation to the eyes of each and every newborn. They were used to prevent gonorrhea, a sexually transmitted disease affecting the mother, from being transferred to the eyes of the baby during the birthing process and causing an eye infection that could cause blindness. The doctors said that such an infection is rare in the United States, but they put in the eye drops anyway. No one thought about it or questioned it because it was routine.

In intermediate care, we calculated all the numbers for the grams of formula, carbohydrates, protein, etc. in the baby formulas. The whole thing was so unnatural. It was as if the professors were saying that the babies were tiny machines that ran on a certain percentage of protein, fat, and carbohydrates with a few vitamins. Women have been breastfeeding since the beginning of time, and I know not all of them have had a college education to even know what carbohydrates are, and yet, they have been able to feed and raise healthy children. In contrast, modern medicine tries to control every single variable of human life, condensing them down to minute facts and details, and then tweaking the details.

We compared cow's milk with soy milk with breast milk and nothing came close to the superiority of breast milk. The cow's milk was especially bad. I can only suppose that it's because cow's milk, genetically speaking, is supposed to be for baby cows, not for baby humans. It grows cows into huge animals, so, of course, the milk contains high amounts of protein and fat. Cow's milk is woefully deficient in iron, and babies develop iron-deficiency anemia if they do not take supplemental iron. The fat content of cow milk is so high that it turns many infants into pudgy, overweight babies.

The research shows that there are a certain number of fat cells made in the beginning years of life, and for the rest of a person's life, those fat cells just get bigger. If a person starts off with a larger number of fat cells, say because they get fat in the first few years of life, then they have a lot more fat cells to fill up during their lifetime. A good reason not to feed cow's milk to human infants.

It seemed like they all should have been on breast milk. In fact, the pediatric professors told us during a study session that they could always tell a baby on cow's milk because they were fat, anemic, and had green snot constantly dripping out of their noses.

The cow protein is foreign to humans and the babies commonly react to it with their immune systems. Their immune systems try to get rid of the milk by producing mucous to protect their cells from the foreign milk protein. It causes runny noses, colds, flu's, ear infections, asthma, eczema, colic and many other conditions. Feeding cow's milk to human babies is like trying to give elephant milk to a baby giraffe; it just doesn't work. The nutrients are not in the right proportions, and there would be foreign proteins that the giraffe would react to in the elephant milk.

I am convinced that the only acceptable food for a baby is breast milk. Even the soy milk formulas gave many babies congestion, but it seemed at least better than the cow's milk. I don't think anyone will ever be able to design a baby formula with the proper proportion of nutrients, antibodies and other components needed for the proper growth and functioning. Scientists are constantly finding new nutrients, vitamins, and antibodies in breast milk that they didn't know existed before. There is no good substitute for breast milk.

Many mothers had been told they could not breastfeed because they were taking a medication that would pass through the breast milk and be toxic to the baby. It seemed logical to assume that a drug toxic to a baby would also be toxic, although less so, to the grownup taking it. I thought, *why were they taking it in the first place?*

Babies not breastfed miss out on all of the protective antibodies that the mother transfers to the baby during the first few days of nursing - it was called colostrum. They also suffered from lack of closeness - lack of the loving touch of their mother during breastfeeding. I watched so many preemies recover so agonizingly slowly when I believed they could have recovered and left the hospital so much more quickly if they had been touched more. There was a research study at the time that came out that showed premature babies healed and matured more quickly when they were touched. Some of these babies were only touched by the nurses and not very often. Sometimes they stayed in the hospital for months with hardly any touching. I wondered how it would affect them as they grew older. Would they be overly fearful, timid, and unsure of themselves because they never had a solid foundation of demonstrative love from the very beginning? Would they turn to a life of crime and drugs due to a lack of self esteem and a lack of belonging? We simply cannot underestimate the power of this bonding that occurs between mother and baby at this crucial time.

Societies who separate their children from their mothers at birth are known to have high rates of violent crime. The United States is one of those societies. It is disastrous and unnatural to separate a baby from its mother right after birth, not only to the child, but also to the family and to the society in which it grows up.

Taking all of this in consideration, adding up the number of the fat grams, and protein and such seemed like a big waste of time to me. These babies and mothers had much bigger problems ahead of them. I thought maybe we should send the babies home with the mothers, get the mothers off of prescription drugs, and send everybody home with herbs so they could breast feed. Maybe I was overly optimistic.

They were just beginning to implement a computerized system whereby we could enter our notes into several computers. We were required to hand write so much on other rotations because doctors were being sued so frequently. It seemed like the practice of medicine was mostly paperwork. Too many tests were ordered to double check their diagnoses. Every minute detail had to be documented concerning what they had told the patients, what procedures they had done, what drugs the patient had been taking, and how exactly the patient had been progressing.

The only downside to the computers was that there were so many computer terminals around so many sick and fragile babies, and the terminals all put out strong electromagnetic fields which had been shown to be harmful, and I knew it was delaying the healing of those babies. It didn't feel right, so much electronic equipment around the sick babies. Computer terminals and other sources of electric fields were all over the hospital. There was actually a hum that I could hear when I entered the intermediate care unit because there was so much electricity coursing through there.

It was interesting that later on in my fourth year, we took a course in epidemiology during which we studied how epidemiologists determine the causes of epidemics. The professor taught us that people living near high power lines had a much higher incidence of brain cancer. It was concluded the electromagnetic field interfered with their brain function.

Not surprisingly, I got a bad cold during this time. Maybe it was all the chemicals I was exposing myself to every day - or maybe the stress. It was also winter time. Claire gave me this herbal formula, and she told me it would make me cough up all the phlegm in my lungs. Lo and behold, the more I took it, the more it made me cough, and the more I coughed out of my lungs until I was well. Instead of the usual five month cough that followed, this one only lasted a few weeks. This was a miracle.

If I had known what I know now, the cold would have only lasted a few days or less. If I had known about juice fasting, garlic and echinacea, and cayenne and hydrotherapy, I could have knocked it out even sooner. As it was, I was taking an echinacea brand that was top of the line, but was compared to the ones I know about now, and even my homemade brews now are several times stronger than what is commercially available. When I make herbs, I mean business. Neither I nor any of my friends are going to the hospital as long as I have herbs as strong as these at home.

The brand I took had so much alcohol in it, and so little echinacea in it that I actually got drunk from taking the doses that Claire recommended. I woke up with a hangover, and I was really furious about it. Since those alcoholic tinctures were not made in the way that makes them strong and not so much alcohol in them, we had to pour boiling water over the dose. That way, the alcohol would evaporate, and we would be left with the herbs only.

One of the other herbs I learned about came from Mexico, and it was regenerating kidneys. Whenever too many toxins were released, they would have to pass through and be processed by my kidneys, and they would be overloaded. When this happened, my urine would become cloudy, and Claire would give me the "Blue water." The "blue water" was made from the bark of a tree. She couldn't get it any other way except to make a trip down to Mexico because they couldn't ship it across the border. It was called blue water because when people made a tea out of it, it was a bluish color. It worked very well, and it did exactly what she said it would do.

All the herbs we need are right near us; we need only look many times in our own backyards for the herbs that will heal us. Although the foreign herbs work well, it's not mandatory for us to go into Mexico or even to China to get some sort of exotic herb to heal ourselves.

But, there were no herbs in Intermediate Care. There were babies that were born to mothers whose Rh blood type was incompatible, causing many complications. They received blood transfusions through their umbilical blood vessels that had not yet closed off. This incompatibility could get so serious that the babies died in the womb. This condition was called fetal hydrops because the babies swelled up with so much fluid. The mother's immune system sees the baby's Rh positive blood cells and hers are Rh negative. The negative factor makes antibodies against the positive and destroys the cells. In Rh incompatibility, the mother's immune cells are killing her baby. To avert this death in the womb and the many complications that could occur at birth, the doctors gave the mother an injection of antibodies to the baby's Rh cells after it was born. It killed off any remaining fetal blood cells in the mother's blood before her immune system could see them and kill them. If her immune system reacted, the rest of the Rh positive babies she would have in the future would be affected.

I used to think this Rh incompatibility could only be treated by giving these injections until I heard about how an herbalist who had both the mother and the father do herbal detoxifying, and change to a natural diet. The mothers had come to him because the medical doctors told them they could no longer have any babies because it was too dangerous. After the detoxifying, they had babies without any complications at all. So many of these abnormal conditions and diseases are caused by an unnatural diet and lifestyle.

I saw was a premature baby born to a mother who had lupus. In people diagnosed with lupus, their immune systems attack their own body. The only thing the doctors knew to do for it was to suppress the immune system by giving steroids. People usually die from lupus. It is characterized by arthritis, fevers, and progressive damage to the kidneys. There can also be inflammation of the heart and lungs. There can be serious problems with the blood like vasculitis, an inflammation of the blood vessels that causes clotting and bleeding, and hemolytic anemia (the immune system destroys the patient's own blood cells). Because of these problems with the blood vessels, it is difficult for the mother's blood vessels to carry good quality blood to the fetus during pregnancy. I was not surprised when the infant, after birth turned out to have a birth defect of the liver. He was the scrawniest baby I ever saw. He had so many problems, he was struggling every minute for survival. The doctors suspected he had biliary sclerosis, a narrowing of the tubules in his liver. For this, he would need a liver transplant, or else he would die.

One does not just get an organ transplant and then live happily ever after. There are problems with rejection and problems with taking drugs that suppress the immune system. There are *serious* life-threatening problems with organ transplants. They do not last forever, either. You don't just get one transplant and keep it the rest of your life. When another transplant is needed, the patient must go through the whole rejection process and hospitalization again, at the cost of several thousands of dollars. Since the insurance pays for it, everyone who pays medical insurance premiums pays for it. What for - so the baby can live for a few more years in and out of a hospital, sick and with a horrible quality of life?

At first glance, we tend to think these surgeries are so wonderful and miraculous, and we do not see them for the horrors that they really can be. We see on the news more brainwashing about how a transplant is such a breakthrough and so important for saving people's lives. We forget to ask, "What are their lives like after the transplant?" We do not see the pain they cause, and don't see the agony of fearing organ rejection. We don't see the big deal about what happens when flu season comes around because anyone on immune suppressing medication is going to succumb to whatever germs are going around, and is going to get it worse and longer or even could die. Most transplants could be avoided if people knew how to heal themselves naturally. I wish I could tell every mother out there to get well before they decide to have babies. The babies with birth defects are not born from healthy mothers. They might be born to mothers whose doctors have told them that they were *basically healthy*. But we all know what that means now. Everyone can get well. Mothers and fathers can prepare themselves to have healthy babies free of birth defects by following a healthy diet and lifestyle and doing some herbal cleansing and detoxification.

There were no herbs or diet changes in the Intensive Care Unit in the next hospital. Every child there was hooked up to tubes of some sort. Some were hooked into a machine that did their breathing for them, or had tubes down their noses into their stomachs to feed them because they couldn't swallow. Some children had all of these. Many of them had cancer.

One of them was there because she had suffered a severe reaction to anesthesia, which had left her paralyzed and almost killed her. She could not breathe on her own, so she was incubated, and she stayed there for weeks struggling for life. Her parents looked on helplessly, not knowing what to do for her, not knowing if what the doctors were doing that particular day was right for her - agonizing over the minute details of her care. She had been on antibiotics to prevent bacterial infections because she had a tube down her trachea that was connected to a machine that breathed for her. Foreign objects such as tubes left in the body for more than a day or so usually become the focal point for an infection.

One day the doctors cultured her sinuses and found fungus. Usually the patients had fungal infections because they had received so many antibiotics that the fungus overgrew. The fungal infection was usually worse than the bacterial infection. The doctors were then going to administer the very toxic antifungal medications. I saw this situation repeatedly in every rotation. First, the bacterial infections and the antibiotics, then the antiviral for the viral infections, then the antifungals for the fungal infection that could eat up half of the face if the doctors couldn't stop it. All the while, their immune systems, which could have fought the infections had they been strong enough, were suppressed from the toxic chemicals being pumped into their bodies every day - from the hospital environment, lack of exercise, and being told constantly that they might not make it. Whatever the original surgery requiring anesthesia, it could have been avoided in the first place with natural healing.

Doctors call the adverse effects from medical treatment iatrogenic disease. For example, one particular heart medication caused lupus-like symptoms and certain antibiotics caused the intestinal lining to slough off, called pseudomembranous colitis. We learned about all sorts of toxic reactions that happened because of medications, like Stevens Johnson syndrome which is a potentially fatal skin rash. It is horribly painful and can be permanently disfiguring, which can result from commonly prescribed antibiotics. I used to take antibiotics all the time for infections. Now that I understand what they can do, and that I can heal with herbs instead, I have not had to take any antibiotics in over 6 years, nor have any of my patients since I switched over to natural methods. Robert Mendelsohn, M.D. noted that most infections he saw usually cleared up on one to two weeks even without antibiotics or any other treatment.

In my second year of school, the professors taught us about bacteriocidal antibiotics and bacteriostatic antibiotics. The bacteriocidal antibiotics killed bacteria and the bacteriostatic ones merely stopped the growth of the bacteria but did not kill it. The professors said it was the patient's own immune system that killed the bacteria even when bacteriocidal antibiotics were administered. The body heals itself; the antibiotics are merely an aid to the body's own miraculous healing power. We should never forget this astounding fact. When we give too many antibiotics, we are actually putting in so many chemicals that we interrupt the body's own way of healing itself. We interrupt the process of the white blood cells attacking and neutralizing the microorganisms. We chemically poison the patient, wondering why we have to keep switching our patients to a different type of antibiotic and why we have to add more antibiotics on to the drug regimen so that people in the hospital are taking up to 4 kinds of antibiotics all at once.

Many people with iatrogenic diseases ended up in the Intensive Care Units. We saw people commonly develop pneumonia as a result of having a tube in their trachea. We saw people commonly get urinary infections from having a catheter in their bladders. We saw people with infections around the place where the I.V's entered into the skin. We saw phlebitis, or inflammation of the veins because of tubes inserted into the blood vessels. We called these infections that people acquired as a result of being in the hospital nosocomial infections. They were common enough for us to have a name for it. More and more I saw the dangerous effects of what medical treatment does to people, and I wanted less and less to become a doctor. It made me more and more not want to ever do these sorts of things to anyone. I saw how much it hurt. I saw how much money was wasted because people had to stay in the hospital longer due to these reactions.

According to the Centers for Disease Control in Atlanta (CDC), a survey of more than 260 hospitals in the U.S. revealed that nosocomial infections have risen sharply in the past 20 years. About 2 million of those infections occurred in 1995 which resulted in around 90,000 deaths. A similar study conducted between 1975 and 1980 showed that the rate had risen 36%. What is of major concern is that as many as 70% of those nosocomial infections were resistant to 1 or more antibiotics. These nosocomial infections cost an extra $4.5 billion per year in health care in the United States. (Source: Emerging Infections on Center Stage at First Major International Meeting, JAMA, April 8, 1998; vol 279, no. 14, p. 1055)

There was another recent study that came out recently in the Journal of the American Medical Association that was shocking because it showed the number of deaths caused by medication reactions to be at least 100,000. They were counting medications that were taken correctly, so these were not expected reactions. They also did not include medications taken with the wrong dose or the wrong frequency, or even mix ups at the pharmacy that caused people to receive the wrong medication entirely. So we can safely assume that many more people are suffering from adverse effects of medications than just what this study found. See study below.

JAMA Reports Drug Errors Costly to Health Care System

Source: American Medical Association Science News press release 1/22/97

According to JAMA studies:

1.   Adverse drug effects (ADE's) rate was 6.5 per hun dred admissions. 28% of these were judged prevent able (!)

2.   The estimated annual additional costs of ADE's occur ring in a large tertiary care hospital were ***$2.8 million***

3.   The estimated annual additional costs associated with all ADE's were ***$5.6 million.***

4   These estimates do <u>not</u> include costs of injuries to pa tients, malpractice costs, or the costs of less serious medication errors or hospital admissions related to ADE's.

5.   The additional length of a hospital stay associated with an ADE was ***2.2 days*** (for a preventable ADE, it was 4.6 days)

6.   The increase in costs associated with an ADE was ***$3,244*** (preventable ADE cost was $5,857.)

7.   They found that the occurrence of an ADE was asso ciated with nearly double the risk of death (1.88).

8.   They found that ADE's may account for up to ***140,000 deaths*** annually in the U.S. placing it some where between the fourth and sixth leading cause of death in the U.S.!!!

Yet another study revealed an estimated one third of drug-related deaths in the emergency department are caused by the abuse or misuse of prescription drugs (*Patient Care.* May 30, 1998, p. 42).

The Alliance for Aging Research has stated in their recent report, "When Medicine Hurts Instead of Helps," that in treating nursing home residents, more money is spent on correcting the health problems caused by drug errors than on the drugs themselves. The elderly are particularly vulnerable to adverse reactions because of the number of drugs they take and because of the biological changes related to aging and disease (Hospital Medicine, 12/98, p. 8). If these drugs are toxic, how is it that they are supposedly "curing" disease?

Another study showed that the pathogens (germs causing diseases) seen in ICU's are changing due to the widespread use of broad-spectrum antibiotics. Between 1992 and 1997, urinary tract infections constituted 31% of nosocomial infections, 27% were due to pneumonia, and 19% were primary bloodstream infections. Invasive devices were associated with the majority of infections in all three major sites: 95% of urinary tract infections (UTI'S) were associated with urinary catheters, 86% of pneumonias were associated with the use of ventilators, and 87% of primary bloodstream infections were associated with central lines - catheters surgically placed in the body to allow a way for the medication to enter directly into a blood vessel.

As we intervene more in the body's natural processes, we will spend much more money. According to recent government projections, spending for healthcare in the United States will double over the next decade, going from $1.035 trillion in 1996 to $2.1 trillion by the year 2007. Spending per person will jump from $3,759 in 1996 to $7,100 in 2007. Projections show Americans will spend much more on prescription drugs, $171 billion in 2007 than the $62 billion spent in 1996 (*Healthcare Spending Expected to Top $2 Trillion*, Physician's Financial News, Oct. 1998, p. 4).

Another one of the patients at the hospital was an 8-year-old boy who was in a coma. It had been one disaster after another. When he was younger, the doctors removed a brain tumor, but the surgery left him with seizures afterwards. The seizure medication helped for a while, and was known to be toxic to the liver. In natural healing, we know that whenever there's a cancer, the liver is not functioning properly, so this was not a good combination. The boy started going into seizures, and the doctors couldn't get him out of it with the regular anticonvulsants. To stop them, they were forced to put him in a drug-induced coma. He had a nasogastric tube through which he was being fed, and he was intubated and on a respirator. A nasogastric tube, also called a feeding tube, is a tube that is inserted through the nose and guided down to the stomach and taped into place. It is used to get foods into the stomach when the patient can't swallow on his own. In this situation, the doctors usually try to get the person out of the coma as soon as possible, but this time it didn't work. Day after day, the resident expressed frustration at her inability to taper him off of the sedating medication that kept him in the coma.

One day, the doctors had ordered a routine X-ray to check the position of the nasogastric tube. It did not end at the proper part of the stomach, so I was asked to assist with repositioning it. When a people are comatose, they have strong reflexes, so that if you try to perform a procedure on them, they will fight you. So, the doctors asked me to hold the child's arm while they repositioned the tube. He started fighting but I was holding him tight. In that moment, I felt so strongly and intensely for him, and I wondered, *why God does he have to go through this? Please help me to help him.* I had no idea what I was doing, but I imagined myself sending him healing energy directly from God. This went on for maybe ten minutes, as it took that long to reposition the tube. I was gripping tightly and praying at the same time - a weird combination.

I didn't think anything about it until the next morning when I came in and the resident was elated. "He's sitting up! He's sitting up today! It's a miracle! He's sitting on the edge of his bed today!" And there he was - a miracle. He continued to improve from that day on. That was my first experience with energetic healing.

The power of love and prayer has no equal. It's said that a person with a disease has a lower frequency than the body of a healthy person, and that there are ways to increase the frequency of a sick person. One of those ways is through love and prayer. We can always benefit from more love in our lives.

I had heard of an herbal formula and also a single herb (lobelia inflata) that many natural healers had used and were still using to successfully stop seizures. Very recently, I had the opportunity to use this formula on a man who was having seizures from alcohol withdrawal. The formula stopped the seizures. Cayenne revived him. It was a miracle. I didn't even have to put him in a coma to stop the seizures.

It was rather anticlimactic. With all of the medical training I had, he didn't have to have any tubes inserted into him or anything else. It was difficult to believe it was that simple. I didn't have the opportunity to use any fancy doctor tools, or even much of my fancy doctor knowledge. Those herbs are God's gifts to us and they are miraculous in what they do.

What I hear and learn from a book or a video is never all the way true to me until I test these things for myself. There is no substitute for experience which is why I don't give much credence to books, especially written by those who have no direct experience with their subject matter. I usually don't pay much attention to the research done on different diseases. My experience always tells me something different. My experience is real and it always wins out over words written by research scientists who, by their own admission, have never "cured" anything.

The rest of the children in the intensive care unit had been diagnosed with RSV – short for Respiratory Syncytial Virus, a very serious virus affecting the lungs. The children required constant medication to keep their lungs open, and sometimes needed to be put on a ventilator because their lungs were so congested and filled with fluid. I could hear the raspy, weak cries from some who were only 4 years old.

There are herbs powerful enough to open up the lungs without the side effects of synthetic medications. Also, a mother could get to the cause of the weak immune system like the child's diet or bowel habits. Remember, I eventually threw out my asthma inhalers and I also threw out my peak flow meter that monitored my breathing capacity. I know this sounds too simple, and again for me to be a trained doctor and not to have to use anything fancy is just a let down. Most of those children wouldn't have been there if everyone understood the principles of natural healing. Taking herbs - (especially echinacea which strengthens the immune system), changing the diet, and eliminating dairy products would have prevented most of these infections. The problem was many mothers are not healthy enough to breastfeed or they're on drugs that are excreted in the breast milk and are too dangerous for a baby to take in that way. If only the mothers would get healthy and take herbs instead, they could all breastfeed their babies. Their babies wouldn't suffer from the toxic effects of synthetic formulas, or worse, pasteurized cow's milk. As I mentioned previously, these things cause excess mucous reactions and asthma, and the chemicals are a strain on the infant's immune system, leading to a condition in the infant's body favorable for the respiratory virus to grow.

One day, I was riding the elevator down to leave the hospital for the day, and I was standing beside a lady with her 4 or 5 year old child in hand. She was saying to another lady that she had just been through hell with the chemotherapy for him, and just when they thought he would recover, the RSV was going around the hospital and he caught it. She referred to the RSV as being the "enemy" that attacked randomly out of the blue. I wanted to tell her it was the chemotherapy that destroyed his immune system so he couldn't fight it off, and probably the sickness had more to do with the child's body trying to eliminate all of the chemicals that had been put into him than it did with a "virus". I also wanted to tell her that it was the *chemotherapy* that was the enemy - not the RSV. Few of us really know what's going on with our bodies and the bodies of our loved ones, so when the doctors say the enemy is the RSV, then we all repeat to our friends and relatives that the enemy is the RSV. She trusted every word they said, as she let them slowly kill her son with more and more chemicals.

Back in the Intensive Care Unit was a 12-year-old girl who had just undergone major surgery on her back. She had been diagnosed with severe cerebral palsy, which resulted in muscles so spastic, they pulled her spine out of alignment - scoliosis. The doctors surgically implanted a rod in her spine to straighten it out. Everything had gone well during the surgery. She came out of surgery in the morning, and in the afternoon, she flat-lined. The whole unit full of medical personnel tried CPR for 4 long hours. I remember everything stopped in the unit while nurses hurriedly opened the sterile equipment needed to inject the I.V. drugs to revive her. They also intubated her, and the students and everyone else not involved stood by and watched. I felt like crying because they were pounding on her chest, and it was so loud, and so violent. First they had sliced open her whole back during the surgery, and now they were pounding on her and sticking needles and tubes into her everywhere. I thought that was just about enough of what a young child could take. None of it did any good. She left us.

Later, I heard a resident say that he hated those spinal surgeries because the risk of death was unacceptably high, and that he had seen many other deaths in the period soon after these surgeries because they were so highly invasive. It took a while to determine the cause of death; she had to be autopsied and I left before we knew the result, but the most likely cause was massive internal bleeding due to the surgery. There is only so much doctors can rip apart a body, and then expect to be able to put it back together again without fatal complications.

There are many antispasmodic herbs and natural healing routines to do for cerebral palsy, and it would have been intense in this particularly severe case, but if she had had these natural healing routines done to the maximum, there would not have been the need for such an invasive back surgery. I know of many deep massage techniques such as Rolfing, which can result in an amazing change in the muscles surrounding the spine. This is only one of many techniques that could have helped her.

The rest of the time I spent on pediatrics was spent in clinic where the children were not quite so sick. There were

192   STOP THE MEDICINE!

new immunization schedules coming out frequently that needed to be committed to memory. Every child got the recommended immunizations. I detested administering them because I had read many works describing their ill effects and their ineffectiveness. I later read Dr. Mendelsohn's <u>Immunizations: The Terrible Truth That Your Doctor Won't Reveal</u>. Dr. Mendelsohn was a prominent medical doctor who served as chief of staff at a major hospital in Chicago and served on the medical licensing board. After so many years of observing what abuses go on in the medical system, he began to speak out. One of the main things he said was that statistically speaking, the odds of surviving are better if people just don't go to the doctor. Doctor visits would result in unneeded procedures or medications which could have some sort of toxic effect that could seriously hurt or kill. He cited studies that showed that when medical doctors went on strike, the death rate actually went down. He was opposed to immunizations as they many times caused the diseases they were supposed to protect against, as well as not providing protection at all, as when the child got the disease anyway. He quoted research showing many immunizations were linked with brain inflammation (meningitis), fevers, uncontrollable crying in children, and learning disabilities later in life.

The new hepatitis vaccine was developed which was supposed to be given to the babies just after birth. During the first two years of school, the professors taught that a baby's immune system was not mature enough to handle immunizations; therefore, a 6-month wait was mandatory before administering their first immunization. Suddenly, we were giving the hepatitis B vaccine at birth when the babies' immune systems were not mature enough to handle it. I felt it was a dangerous thing to do, especially considering what they had previously taught us. They offered no explanation as to why it was suddenly safe to vaccinate babies at birth; it was just an order handed down that had to be followed. Like good sheep, we followed, and all the patients followed us - they were good sheep, too and didn't question us.

Later on, I learned during a pathology rotation that the first hepatitis B vaccines were obtained from the blood of hepatitis patients, many of whom had AIDS and other diseases. Vaccines rarely can be sterilized sufficiently to contain only the one part of the disease that they are designed to prevent. Usually, the vaccines are taken from animals or humans infected with the virus or bacteria in question. The problem is that animals and humans don't just have that one particular type of organism in their bodies at any given moment – they can have several, maybe hundreds of different types of disease-causing organisms in their bodies at any given moment.

I believe it is impossible to isolate one particular organism and put it into a vaccine. What we end up with is a vaccine that we think is pure, isolated and sterile, until we develop new, more powerful microscopes. To our horror, we have discovered that there are hundreds of other organisms in the vaccine that we did not have the technology to see when we first made it. This is why the recent polio virus was recalled. It was contaminated with microorganisms other than the polio virus. I do not possibly think that putting other peoples' and animals' infected secretions into our bodies is going to make us healthy, or keep us from getting sick. With all of these fluids and blood used to make vaccines, they certainly are not kosher, nor are they healthy.

I moved on to pediatric neurology where I interviewed lots of children with seizures. They were spaced out like zombies, which was probably caused by a combination of their seizures not being adequately controlled by the medication, and the medication effects themselves. I swore I'd never take that medication, and I never did. I always would check their blood tests for liver damage, as it was standard procedure to check for patients who took medications that could potentially cause toxic effects on the liver, which was called drug-induced hepatitis. If there was liver damage, the doctors were supposed to switch the patient to a different drug. By that time, however, there had already been damage done. People suffering from the effects of liver-damaging medications might notice that they've lost energy and their sex drive, they've caught more colds and flu's, and they've started forgetting things frequently and maybe they've developed Alzheimer's disease. Then they might get a cancer. They might have developed cancer, thinking it had nothing to do with the medication because the doctor told them if they saw any damage done, they would stop the medication - well, *obvious* damage, that is. Obvious damage shows up on the blood tests while subtle damage usually does not.

They assumed the medication was safe. Doctors thought thalidomide was safe, too, but now we know that when pregnant ladies take it, their babies are born with severe deformities like missing arms. Diethylstilbesterol (DES) was considered safe, and they used it to prevent miscarriages. Yet, they found out later that it caused the children to grow up with severe defects of the reproductive system like a deformed uterus and vaginal cancer. Fen-phen was also considered safe until the FDA reviewed echocardiographic evidence that showed heart valve abnormalities in 31% of the patients tested (Source: Food and Drug Administration. *FDA Analysis of Cardiac Valvular Dysfunction With Use of Appetite Suppressants.* Rockville, Md: Division of Pharmacovigilance and Epidemiology, Food and Drug Administration, US Dept of Health and Human Services; 1997). They thought it was safe...doesn't take a genius to figure out that when they say that... Discovering new dangers of drugs after marketing evidently is common, according to the U.S. General Accounting Office. Overall, 51% of approved drugs had serious adverse effects not detected prior to approval by the FDA (Source: US General Accounting Office, *FDA Drug Review: Postapproval Risks, 1976-85.* Washington, DC: US General Accounting Office; April 26, 1990. GAO/PEMD-90-15). If that weren't enough, consider that each year prescription drugs injure 1.5 million people so severely they require hospitalization and 100,000 die, making prescription drugs a leading cause of death in the United States (Source: Lazarou J, Pomeranz BH, Corey PN. Incidence of adverse drug reactions in hospitalized patients: a meta-analysis of prospective studies. *JAMA*. 1998;279:1200-1204).

Once again, after being questioned on my own condition during this rotation, I mentioned that I saw a nutritionist, and was told that this was a very dangerous thing to do, and that I must see a "real" doctor. Silly me, maybe I was just imagining my recovery, because after all, this "quackery" was allowing me to heal enough to keep going to medical school so that I could hear all of my peers tell me how they thought I was hurting myself with natural healing.

Family Practice

Play With Drugs To Get Burned

Family Practice was at the Cody White clinic again. There were so many people there. I was mesmerized by the sheer number walking to and fro just inside the main entrance. I couldn't believe so many people could be sick and taking synthetic chemicals into their bodies.

Family practice was a little different because the doctors actually were telling us to try to figure out the reason the patient was sick. They lectured to us on the importance of the family unit and the community, and they wanted us to ask all of these questions. When it came down to it, no one wanted the students to spend too much time with the patients, so there was a lot of talk that was hardly ever implemented.

I very much disliked learning the minor surgical procedures. One of the common procedures involved removing part of the toenail when it was ingrown. This was more complicated than it sounded. It could be a bloody mess. In fact, the portion of the toenail I removed during my first procedure wouldn't stop bleeding. I think it had something to do with how much alcohol the teenage boy drank. In large amounts, alcohol suppresses the body's ability to make platelets that are responsible for clotting the blood. We commonly saw this in alcoholics.

The attending physician told me to elevate the boy's foot, continuing to apply direct pressure until the bleeding stopped. It didn't. A routine procedure. There's no such thing - every day I went into the hospital, I kept getting more confirmation of this fact. Even the easiest of procedures could turn into a complicated mess. I sat and sat and sat, holding this young man's toenail which kept oozing blood. The attending kept yelling at me as if it were my fault the toenail was still bleeding, and that I must hurry up with this case so I could go on and see other patients. Finally, it stopped, but not before the attending had yelled at me so many times for taking so long that I never wanted to see his face again. He kept reminding me that there were more patients to see. I didn't think it fair to leave a patient in the middle of bleeding just so that I could go see another patient. The attending wanted to herd the patients in, and herd the patients out. And in between, if I wrote a 2 minute prescription or did a 5 minute procedure, that would be fine. But don't mess up the way we do things here, young lady, was what he really seemed to be communicating.

Then there were the dressings. One patient came in to have a dressing changed. He had had a skin infection on his face that turned into a large pocket of pus that one of the doctors had previously lanced open to get the pus out. He was another alcoholic who had an infection because the alcohol suppressed his immune system, that made it more likely to get infections of all kinds. The doctor had packed it with gauze, and bandaged it up to be changed by someone else at this date. The resident asked me to change it, yet I had no idea how to conduct such a procedure. As usual, she quickly disappeared right after she gave the order without seeing if I knew what I was doing. There was rarely enough supervision. Sometimes I had to sit there and wait because I couldn't just start guessing and working on patients. As if I were going to start digging around in this man's wound without knowing what I was doing! By the time the resident or attending came back, they'd be yelling again because I was taking so long. Catch-22.

The resident halfway showed me how to change the

dressing and repack the wound, but not without giving me a stern lecture about how incompetent I was that I didn't know how to do it. None of the other students knew how to do it, either. She demonstrated the techniques, as if she really did not want me to learn how to do it, as if she really didn't care if I learned it, and she really didn't care to be there at all. I didn't believe she liked working there. She had that typical attitude that sometimes develops during medical training - you just don't care, and you start to hate your patients and everyone around you. She happened to be pregnant, and my guess was that she was barely making the demands of her work with all of the sleep deprivation and having to deal with a pregnancy at the same time.

I myself was constantly being hurried along as I tried to fulfill the requirements that had been set forth. Again, the Catch-22. We were trying to ask questions many times of patients who didn't understand the importance, or who just said outright, "That's not important! Where's the real doctor?" Some of them would yell at me for not following the system - they didn't want me to ask about their life. They just wanted to have their prescription written and be on their merry way. They had been well-trained by the doctors to get in and out by their doctors to get in and out of the office quickly. They didn't want to know why they were sick - that was just a random event that came out of the blue and struck them because they were unlucky victims. They just wanted their "magic" pill, so they could go about their business, not knowing they were getting sicker and sicker and sicker over the years, and continuing to return to the clinic.

It was like some sort of sick ritual. Everyone went through the motions without really knowing why. The patients kept returning because we kept taking out and destroying parts of their bodies. They would require prescriptions for life. We would irradiate their thyroids - killing the thyroid so that it made no thyroid hormone at all, so they would need to take the synthetic hormone for the rest of their lives. It would keep them coming into the doctors over and over again. We

would tell them that they needed hormone replacement therapy - again, it kept them coming back. We kept the diabetics
coming back for years for their magic "sugar-lowering" pills
and insulin.

They kept coming back for the antibiotics because
their infections kept coming back. The same kind of infections they had had before would come back, and a major reason being that they had never cured the infection in the first
place with the antibiotics. They had never cleaned out the old
mucous in their sinuses, the same mucous that the viruses and
bacteria thrived on. They never coughed out the accumulated
putrefied material in their lungs that caused them to have repeated episodes of asthma and pneumonia and bronchitis. All
these conditions could have been healed with herbs. They
never learned how to clean out their colons, so they kept coming back for the immune-suppressing medications to keep the
colitis symptoms under control. They continued the gout
medication instead of changing their diets and detoxifying
their bodies. Maybe if someone had told them they had the
chance of being totally well, they would have made lots of
changes and would have been willing to try natural methods.

Most of the problems we saw were complications
from drinking alcohol, smoking, overeating and taking recreational drugs. I supposed I should qualify that illness caused by
prescription drugs was common, also. So many times, I would
hear a resident or an attending physician yell out that some incompetent doctor had allowed this patient to be placed on too
many medications, and they were interacting with each other,
making the patient ill. It was always someone else's fault.
Doctors tend to not only blame their patients for being sick,
but to blame each other for the patient being sick. I guess
someone has to take the blame, because doctors really don't
know why the patient is sick in the first place. Blaming makes
disease and control seem under our control if it allows us to
explain why they are happening. It's too threatening to think
that the entire system of medicine, for the most part, doesn't
work.

There was literally a quagmire of drug samples in all of the cabinets. We gave them out like candy. The newest drug would come out, and we'd get a brief comment about it, usually from a resident who only knew about it because he had just heard about it from a drug representative. The most common were the pain relievers, since almost every patient was taking them. So many had pain and arthritis, and since there is no known medical cure for these "illnesses," everyone with a painful condition took pain medication every day. Then we were taught that people taking analgesics every day, especially the nonsteroidal inflammatory medications (called NSAID's for short) would commonly get kidney damage. It could be dangerous if elderly people took too much acetaminophen because they could accidentally overdose and put themselves into liver failure. Lots of people have healed themselves of arthritis with natural methods. The worse thing that happens if someone overdoses on an herb is that he vomits - I would take that any day over liver or kidney damage.

I saw many patients, and we were supposed to keep scheduling their patients for follow-up visits so that we could track their disease. They would come in so fatigued and so chronically ill, I sometimes wondered, how does a person deal with a chronic disease for so many years? I saw one lady with heart disease who had repeated lapses of congestive heart failure with chronic swelling of her legs and ankles, and she didn't complain one time. In fact, she blessed me, complimented me and hugged me when we were finished with the visit. I had so much guilt that day because I didn't want to risk telling her what I knew about natural healing so that she could get some relief. She had such a good attitude, I figured maybe God was probably taking care of her, even in her infirmity. Sometimes people are a lot stronger than we give them credit for. I always found that when patients had a strong faith or belief, that they recovered much faster from surgeries, side effects, and procedures. They were the only ones who seemed to survive the deadly chemotherapy. Their minds were so strong that they were going to stay on this planet and get done what they wanted to get done.

I knew the power of my **own** mind had to be un-
leashed in order to heal myself, so I started working on my
own attitude. I began forgiving everyone in my past who I
thought had wronged me. I looked at my health program as a
gift and a miracle to me. I saw the carrot juice as giving me
extra days of life. I thanked God for giving me the opportunity to experience life for one more day. I stopped to smell
the roses, and anything else beautiful in my path, and practiced gratefulness for the small things. Soon, I stopped expecting everything and everyone to be perfect as I had expected. This was very difficult because I had blamed myself
and everyone around me for everything bad that had ever happened in my life. Eventually, I realized that no one is ever at
fault; life just is.

It was hard to let go of the perfect details - the point
of being a doctor is knowing the minutiae and the research
perfectly. When everyone started to quote the research, I simply tuned out. Instead, I tuned into the birds singing, the
crickets at night, and fully feeling my lover's arms around me.

If you listen to the words of a dying person, they will
tell you that they would have lived their life more fully. They
would have taken more vacations, had more fun and taken off
more time from work. I didn't want to live the rest of my life
with regrets at the end, so I decided to live as fully as I could
in each moment - no regrets.

I realized there was more about me than my rote ability to repeat random facts. One of the reasons I went to
medical school was so that I would appear smart. I wanted
people to listen to me and to think I had something important
to say. And all of those random facts – they were going to
convince everyone how wonderful I was because the truth was
that I, like most people, have no idea what self-love really is. I
couldn't accept that I was wonderful without "being somebody" - somebody considered brilliant, intelligent, at the top
of my field, or beautiful by *everyone else but myself.* I had to stop
trying so hard to "be somebody" and learn how to be myself

for the first time.

I had no idea who I was or what I wanted out of my life. It was like I was living out the expectations of everyone around me, and I had never paid close attention to what *I* wanted. The great thing about the disease was that it really woke me up. I had the chance to discover who I was and what I wanted. The best thing is, I'm still discovering it.

But people get sick for a big reason: because it's time to move on to the next very different part of their lives, and experiencing this sickness is the only way they're going to change. I never would have made so many changes in my life if I hadn't been so severely ill - there would have been no reason to. If life is going along so wonderfully, why change it? The miracle of being human is that we strive so hard to overcome obstacles. We do all sorts of impossible things in order to be whole again.

Sometimes we don't understand it's not that we want to heal our disease, it's really that we want to heal our lives - we want to have peace and love and understanding and acceptance, especially of ourselves. We listen to all of the voices of disapproval and criticism from childhood on from everyone and everywhere. We hear it on TV, on the radio, and in the newspaper that we have to be a certain way or we won't be accepted, and we believe it. We believe we're supposed to live up to the romantic fantasies in the commercials, on billboards, and in magazines all created in the minds of advertising personnel designed to sell a product. So many products are sold due to our insecurities. We listen to women berate their bodies only to have their unsightly problem solved by liposuction, surgery, dieting, implants, or other procedures. But, we never think that our entire society is based on the fact that no one unconditionally loves himself. This lack of self-love has caused and contributed to so much disease. The bottom line was that I had to learn to accept myself exactly as I was - sick and all. I had to love myself even with the possibility that I could be sick the rest of my life.

Sometimes patients would come in with their lives so

devastated by disease that I would have to just give it up to the faith that somehow everything was supposed to be happening exactly this way for very good reason. That helped. What really bothered me was that I was beginning to make decisions regarding patient care that involved looking up the particular medication to administer and in what dose, and then writing out the orders in the chart. My notes always had to be co-signed by a licensed doctor, so technically the responsibility was not mine, and I took some comfort in that. I knew that under different circumstances, for most of the patients, I wouldn't have given them the drugs at all. I'd have told them to detoxify their bodies and change their attitude, food choices and exercise routine, as well as to do some emotional healing.

One lady came into the clinic with multiple psychiatric diagnoses. She had hallucinations, and was depressed. She had had problems for years for which she was solely under the care of a psychiatrist. Since she was diagnosed with a mental disorder, she never went to a regular doctor for her physical health, only the psychiatrist. Doctors tend to see diseases as only one or the other - mental or physical and just care for that one aspect. The only reason she came into the clinic is that for some reason, after all those years, her psychiatrist decided to check her vitamin B12 level. It was extremely low, and the physical exam confirmed. She had a severe vitamin B12 deficiency that had been causing all of her psychiatric symptoms for so long. While the teaching doctor tried to go through the particular test with me, to determine the exact cause of the deficiency, I tried to imagine what her life had been like - being treated like a mental case when she had a severe vitamin deficiency. What irony. I saw many patients in the same situation. While I tried to learn what the Schillings test was to diagnose her, the doctor was talking about treatment as if it were something detached and routine. Injections with high doses of vitamin B12 for a while, and then a maintenance dose for the rest of her life would simply take care of it. She would come in for the shot, and in five minutes, she would be out the door again. If she has any mental problems, that's not for us to deal with, but for the psychiatrist. God forbid she be angry at having been misdiagnosed all of those years.

So I ordered the test done and rescheduled her for another visit. She returned promptly because we had such good rapport. I remember that day because it was raining hard, which meant that most patients didn't show up for their visits. But she did. The laboratory messed up repeatedly and I never got to the exact cause for her deficiency - pernicious anemia, malabsorption, bowel cancer, etc. It was a struggle to get anything done since many of the clinic employees didn't want to do their jobs, and so the most routine tests took forever. I wondered how was her life during these periods between visits? As her life was put on hold by the expectation of finding out what was causing her disease, she appeared not to care. Her mind was so far gone, there was too much deterioration of her nervous system, and I was told by the doctors that the nervous system damage caused by B12 deficiency was considered irreversible. She could no longer prepare a simple meal for herself.

Sometimes I would just sit and talk with the patients about their lives if they would let me, and if it was a slow enough day that I could get away with it. I saw less patients, but I learned more. I learned more not necessarily about disease but about the way it affects peoples' lives. I wanted to know what it was like for them to be sick. Some of them enjoyed it and some felt awful, and some of them suffered horribly and also wanted everyone to know about it so they could get attention. Some felt awful but didn't want anyone to know about it because they felt like such a burden. Some considered it a minor temporary inconvenience, while others got angry, yelled and blamed the doctors and everyone else.

I saw all degrees of anger, hopelessness, despair, resignation, and acceptance of disease, and it fascinated me. The alcoholics and drug addicts were angry and full of blame while the cancer patients were sweet and never said much; they just let everyone walk all over them like doormats without a peep.

Some of them sighed and said things like, "It's God's will", so they figured there was nothing that could be done about their condition. I never was very good at walking away from a patient after asking the "required" questions - I always wanted to know more. Just couldn't help myself I guess - there was too much to know about people. There was a human being in the chair sitting across from me wanting me to help them, and how could I just sit there like a robot asking empty scientific questions when it was their life that brought them there - not necessarily their disease.

My superiors rated me as being very thorough. They thought I was taking so much time because I wanted to get all the details down. I really wanted to know all the reasons why they were sick and why they were there. Some people came in not necessarily because they were that sick, but because they were lonely and because they just wanted someone to listen. I wondered, why is this person coming in for such a minor problem? Then I realized that they wanted someone to listen because no one else in their life would. It seems so easy to listen to someone, but when we really think about it, how many times do we listen to our friends' problems and interrupt with what we think they should do before they even say they want an answer? Maybe they don't want an answer; maybe they just want us to listen and say that we believe in their ability to work it out. Maybe we've forgotten reassurance and loving someone exactly the way they are despite their weaknesses.

In the old days, doctors used to be involved in the lives of their patients, they would take time to talk and ask about not just the patient, but the patient's family and job as well. Nowadays, the average office visit only allows enough time for a quick statement of the problem, a few seconds of listening to the heart with a stethoscope and sending the patient off to the laboratory for blood tests.

In the first two years of school, the professors used to teach us that 95% of the time, a doctor should be able to figure out the diagnosis just by taking a thorough history, asking pertinent questions, and doing a good physical exam. Now, it seems the trend has reversed itself. Instead of relying on our clinical judgment, we rely on blood tests. We have distanced ourselves from patients by the overuse of laboratory tests. What we're finding is that the rate of correct diagnosis continues to decrease as we continue to try to automate the diagnostic process. Yet life is the mysterious, delicately complex, wonderful, mind-boggling process that cannot ever be quantified by a lab test or a mathematical equation.

When learning anatomy and physiology, we understood how all of the organs worked, yet something mysterious remained. Who or what told them to work? That's fine that there are these chemical reactions taking place in the body, but what starts and sustains those reactions? What is it we really want to know when we study the human body? Are we trying to find our souls? Soul-searching is a personal, individualized process - it cannot be commercialized. It cannot be quantified with a number; it cannot be researched, and it cannot be dissected. Many may not even have words for their feelings. They are unable to label their feelings as anger, fear, frustration, joy, sorrow, grief - they just start yelling. Can you give me the exact quantifiable reason you feel happy on a warm day when the sun hits your face and there is ever so slight a breeze? How do we think that our physical bodies, the workings of which may be infinitely more complex than our feelings, can be described with a series of numbers? I hope no one thinks that life is all about what the blood test says. I really don't care what the tests say. I care about my patients' lives - this is more important.

What we're really afraid of is that we really don't understand the first things about life or why we even exist. In order not to be too scared about it, we figure if we can just quantify life in terms we can understand, it would ease our anxiety; it would make life predictable. It would also take away the excitement, the spontaneity, and wanton abandon, leaving out love, hope, joy, fear, and anger. It would leave out those wonderful feelings we as doctors feel when a patient tells us something funny or useful or about a personal detail in their life like their new child, their new girlfriend, their new job and so on. It would leave out the satisfaction of knowing that you've done your best to help someone, that it worked and they appreciate you. It would never reproduce that caring that you feel when your patient is a wonderful human being and you know they're doing their best to live their lives, too.

Then there is the whole issue of laboratory errors. A person is not the summation of the particular levels of elements in his blood at a particular frozen nanosecond of time. A cholesterol level does not a personality make. Sedimentation rate tells us nothing about the person's dreams, passions, and talents. It doesn't tell us why the person is depressed. The test knows nothing about a person's life. It won't tell us that the patient's blood pressure is high because they don't exercise, drink enough water, and because their boss and their spouse stress them out. It doesn't tell us the reason for the high cholesterol could be that the patient is so depressed about a divorce that they've been overeating on high fat foods to comfort themselves ever since.

A lab test tells you nothing about a person's self esteem, nothing about their attitudes, and nothing about their motivation to heal (some do not want to heal), or their potential to heal. A lab test does not tell you the exact moment a person will die. Even the prognosis given is merely a doctor's estimation. It doesn't tell you that a big reason the heart is diseased is because the person years ago truly loved someone, lost them, and has closed off their heart to ever loving again in order to avoid the pain of it.

So, I always talked to my patients. There was a particular lady who came into the office of a doctor under whom I was doing a preceptorship. She had a severe skin disease called pemphigus vulgaris. Since it was a rare condition, even after years of practicing, the doctor had to look it up to know what it was. He went through the whole routine of telling her what to do for it, never asking her what she thought about it. Later she told me that she had been experimenting with herbs. But the herbs she had tried were processed and encapsulated -

- horrible quality. She also mentioned that she had a friend who could get her fresh chaparral, and asked if I thought that would do anything. I told her it was a very powerful blood and lymph cleanser, and then asked her what she thought about it, and what did she want to do? She never came back for the follow-up visit. That was her answer - she took the herbs.

I really enjoyed this preceptorship since I got to see the "stuff" the family practitioner was made out of. When an elderly man came in complaining that he had fallen in the shower and hurt his finger, the doctor shot some X-rays and determined that the finger was dislocated. It was fairly obvious - the finger was bent in an unnatural way. The doctor forced the finger back into position. Easier said than done. There was screaming and wailing, the likes of which are only heard in doctor's offices and hospitals, but the finger was finally fixed. I wondered if I would ever have enough guts to work on a man's finger while he was screaming like that.

Family practice got to be routine because most everyone came in with the same problem: allergies and sinus infections. In fact, the doctor had a protocol for it - a certain decongestant, a penicillin derivative antibiotic, and a steroid shot. They all went away with relief. But, they all came back with the same problem 6 months later. Nothing is "cured" with chemicals. The problem is merely forced into suppression temporarily.

It may be shocking, but the number of antibiotic prescriptions in the U.S. is about 3 times the number of prescriptions per person in countries with the best antibiotic prescribing practices, such as Sweden and the Netherlands. Antibiotic prescription rates are not falling, despite warnings that microbes are becoming increasingly resistant. Nonhospital pharmacies in the Unites States are dispensing more antibiotics than ever, based on 1992-1996 data obtained by IMS Health, a pharmaceutical research organization. The number of prescriptions written per year ranged from nearly 267 million to more than 291 million (Source: Antibiotic Prescription Rates

Hold Steady Despite Warnings; *Internal Medicine News*, Nov. 11, 1998, p. 26).

Eighty per cent of all persons seeking medical attention for respiratory illnesses are treated with antibiotics even though pneumonia is considered the only infection for which antibiotics are almost always appropriate. Pneumonia occurs in only 2% of all respiratory illnesses, and more than half of the cases of ear infections, sinus infections, and sore throats are caused by a virus. Viruses are not killed by antibiotics. Antibiotics stop the growth of and kill bacteria, but not viruses. It is estimated that 33 million unnecessary prescriptions for antibiotics are written every year at a cost of over $300 million. According to one study, the excessive use of antibiotics in doctors' offices has contributed to the emergence and spread of antibiotic-resistant bacteria, in particular, Streptococcus pneumoniae. Strep pneumoniae is the leading cause of meningitis, blood infections, and community-acquired pneumonia in this country and is also responsible for about 50% of ear infections in children. The study stated that in adults and children, the strongest and most consistent risk factor for infection was the prior use of antibiotics (Source: Antibiotic Resistance and Prescribing Practices, *Hospital Practice,* April 15, 1998, p. 11-12).

According to the Centers for Disease Control, the estimate for unnecessary prescriptions is even higher, estimated at 50 million, which includes 17 million written for the common cold (also caused by viruses for which antibiotics do not work)

With all of these prescription drugs going around, I was not surprised to see many pharmaceutical representatives at the family practitioner's office. They made regular visits to give their spiel and leave their free samples. Not so long ago, the drug reps would even offer doctors free trips and expensive gifts for prescribing their brand of drugs. Nowadays, the medical profession has put a cap on the monetary value of the gifts allowed.

There was one particular drug rep, a very well-dressed lady who sauntered into the office one day oozing with sex appeal, saying in a somewhat childish sexy voice, "You are prescribing _____ for your patients, aren't you?" She might as well have flipped her fancy pleated short skirt up or taken off her perfectly pressed blouse. Maybe that's what made her a good drug rep. The male doctor replied that of course he was. The way she pranced about with that perfect perky smile reminded me of a Barbie doll. She left more free samples after educating him for about 5-10 minutes on the drug - its dose, side effects, indications, etc. I think her spiel was the only information he ever got about the new drugs that came out. Good thing she came by. The funny thing was that she was not a medical doctor; what made her the authority on treating patients? How did she know if her drug would help his patients? She was earning money for her company by getting as many doctors as possible to write prescriptions for that particular brand drug.

We could always tell the drug reps because they were the best-dressed people in the office and in the hospitals. Many of my friends would seek them out because they knew they had free gifts and sample medications, and they wanted free drugs (sounds a little sick to me) My friends abused this privilege of getting free samples, and always took medication for the slightest ill because it was free and so available.

There were so many drugs that a doctor couldn't keep up with them (new ones came out so frequently), and it was standard practice to have several reference books handy to look up the drugs, their dose, interactions, etc. It was the medical students who really understood the newest drugs the best solely because they had just finished studying them.

A family came in to the clinic with their daughter who had severe abdominal pain. The family doctor decided it was appendicitis, and sent her directly to surgery where the appendix was removed. I thought it a strange coincidence because the father was wearing a hat that said something about steaks, and as it turned out, he sold them for a living. It didn't take me long to figure out that they were feeding their daughter lots of steak, constipating her and causing the appendicitis which put her life in danger. Advanced constipation causes appendicitis. The pressure that builds up in a constipated colon presses fecal matter into the appendix and causes appendicitis.

I remember during my first two years of school, we students watched a film entitled, "Twenty Causes of An Acute Abdomen," in other words, the 20 causes for an abdominal emergency, mostly requiring surgery. It showed how meat and gristle and even buckshot would become lodged in the intestines, in the stomach, in the appendix - anywhere in the intestines. I didn't want to eat meat anymore after I saw that film. There were other causes of an acute abdomen, like an infected gallbladder, but none were so vivid as the gristle in the guts and bones in the meat that were inadvertently swallowed. It drove home the point that meat is very difficult to digest. There were no pictures of vegetables or fruits stuck in the intestines - only meat.

By this time, I had seen so many people with high cholesterol levels and having so many other problems caused by eating meat, that I started recommending everyone become a vegetarian. Unfortunately, they didn't do what I said because the doctor came in right after me with a weight loss restricted calorie diet that included meat and other animal products. Obviously, he had seniority, so they all listened to him. At least he was telling them to lose weight. I had heard of natural healers and even medical doctors who had placed their patients on pure vegetarian diets, and their cholesterol levels fell to normal in one month. I had become a vegetarian again at that time, despite the fact that Claire had told me in the beginning that I had to eat meat to stimulate my adrenals which were so weak. I felt much better without the meat.

After spending over twenty years at her clinic, Claire told me she wanted to retire and do some traveling. She kept telling me that she wanted to hand over her clinic to someone who knew what they were doing, and since I was getting all of this great medical training, she wanted me to be the one. But, every time I asked her about the why's and how's of her treatment programs, she would clam up or say very little. I wanted to know everything there was about healing. I was too impatient to wait for occasional tidbits of knowledge - this was important!

There was a piece of mail I received one day from a man describing the successful natural treatment of serious diseases. For some reason, it was different from the other herbal junk mail I had been receiving - you know, the "Lose weight in 5 days, arthritis pain gone in seconds," and my favorite, "Dreaded disease gone after taking famous European formula!." No, this particular letter talked about detoxifying -- everything that I had already been doing and which I knew worked. I began to subscribe and to inform myself even more. I wanted to know what to do naturally for everything, not just the minor conditions. In time, I began to understand herbalism and natural healing in a way that would allow me to know what to do in just about every situation from the most simple to the most life-threatening with solely natural healing techniques. I learned that there were herbs that were antispasmodic that would have stopped my seizures (I had had to go through them as I was healing them). I learned that Claire was not the only intense natural healer out there. I began to collect all of the information I could, spending a lot of money in the process on videos and books. I've never regretted it. I was investing in my future as a natural healer. I had a clinic ready and waiting for me when I was finished with my medical training. What more could I ask for?

The newsletters described the causes of disease as malnutrition (yes - especially in the United States due to refined foods!) emotional, lack of exercise, lack of circulation, toxic colon, toxic liver, toxic kidneys, and a toxic bloodstream. They were full of very intense routines used for healing oneself of pretty much every disease out there that traditional medical doctors would consider incurable.

By that time I wasn't at all surprised to hear about the miracles that happened when people cleansed the old, accumulated wastes and poisons from their bodies and changed their lifestyle. By now, I had come to see those sorts of healing miracles as ordinary events.

I began to order very powerful herbs and I played around with them, although I have to admit that I was afraid of trying anything on my own, because I was so dependent on my nutritionist for every detail of my illness.

The major problem I had in overcoming the seizures was that I was too dependent. I was looking at natural healing as if it were Western medicine when it couldn't be farther from it. Natural healing, I would learn, was finding the real doctor inside, not looking for it elsewhere and hanging on other experts' words, but very deeply looking inside oneself and having the courage to face one's own demons – in my case, to ask myself why I fell ill in the first place, and to do whatever modifications in my healing program that I felt would be necessary for a healing. I had to stand up and say, "I'm here in this life, and this is what I plan to do with it. I'm making my own decisions from now on, and I trust myself to make the ones that will help me." This was the most difficult lesson I ever learned. I had been looking to my nutritionist for every dosage change, and she was very good about taking charge of that - her word was gospel. Everyone was too afraid to vary by a millimeter from what she had recommended. And so was I.

I had already experienced the nightmare of what this sort of mentality can create, having spent some time in a nursing home taking care of a few patients. The patients were so drugged on so many different types of medications that they couldn't think straight. They had become docile, compliant, and didn't ask any questions. As a result, they were slowly wasting away - slowly dying from the poisons that the doctors put into their bodies every day. They did whatever they were told.

Personally, I think we should make it our goal in life to challenge and to question everything. What is the point of going through life just passively accepting what everyone tells us is the truth? What is the truth? We should go, ask questions and find out! Or we could just rot on our couches watching hours and hours of television and never change our daily routines.

After months of doing Claire's intense cleansing and healing program, I finally got a reward for my healing efforts. Without realizing it, I had run to my car for something because I was in a hurry. I RAN to my car. When I got there, I realized that I RAN. I RAN; I didn't just walk with great weakness, I ran - only for a minute, but I ran! God bless this wonderful planet that we live on - everyone gets a second chance! I'm going to make it! I'm getting my second chance! I loved running, and as a teenager, had run many races. All at once, I began to feel very powerful.

From then on, it didn't seem to matter when my classmates made fun of me. Really nothing else mattered except finishing getting well, so I blocked everyone out so as not to give them a chance to tell me once again not to follow this crazy program recommended by a dangerous quack. They could all go to la-la land for all I cared. This healing was about me, and there was no way I was stopping now.

I'm so fortunate that I had the chance early on in my life to learn how to get and stay healthy because now I won't have to learn it all at once when I am 70 years old and in a nursing home or dying of a rapidly-growing cancer. Maybe I could have done it, but there are some times when it really is just too late. Over the years after medical school, I had tried to help elderly people in nursing homes. It always turned out the same way. The nurses weren't willing to follow the herbal instructions, and the diet was so horrible at those homes that eating was only making them sicker. It wasn't unless a relative brought in decent food and juices and herbs and administered it themselves that the patients experienced any results. It was so frustrating to know the natural methods worked, but yet not be able to implement them because the system was so rigid. It did not seem that nursing homes were about getting people well; they were about stashing people away with the least amount of trouble. The occupants were so senile and so sick that they didn't even realize they were getting poor care. They were so overmedicated I swore they were senile from their medication and that they were dying from overmedication. It seemed as if everyone just wanted the patients to be quiet and not make a fuss. After seeing this, I promised myself I would get and stay healthy right now and for the rest of my life.

Before the days of refined foods and contaminated meat, people lived into their old age with scarcely any disease. There was no arthritis, no senility - only a gradual slowing down. These people died in their sleep without a major fanfare of heart monitors, drugs, and CPR. They just died because it was their time, not because of a disease. Disease results from violating the laws of nature - wrong food choices, wrong attitude, wrong exercise habits, too much stress, and not enough connection to the planet. Aging does not mean one has to get a disease. Considering that every day I am healthier than the day before, I'd say I was on my way to a vital, healthy old age. I will have old age where before there would have been none. So fortunate I was to have lived at all.

When my peers used to express concern that I was playing with dangerous quackery while delaying much-needed medical attention, I learned how to say, "Thanks for being concerned." Then I shut my mouth and said nothing further. It was hard. I wanted to say more. But I had to draw the line, be short, and be firm. I also learned how to take one sentence out of what people would say, find some truth in it, and agree with them on that particular point. This would give them the impression that I agreed with them about everything, and I went on my merry way, not mentioning it to them again, but still doing everything I needed to do with my healing. Tricky? Manipulative? Maybe, but it saved my life. Sure, I would have wanted their support, but they weren't going to give it to me if I told them everything about what I was doing, and I would rather have *not* had their support than to have had their active resistance.

I learned that if I had any doubt about what I was doing, that people would pick up on that and feel they needed to give me advice to help me. I learned that if I told everyone I was handling it, and I was feeling fabulously great - that I didn't care if I turned orange from the carrot juice, and that in fact I enjoyed it because I didn't look so pale anymore - that people wouldn't butt in so much with their opinions. I knew they didn't understand. I knew medicine had no idea what a real healing was. I tried not to hold it against anyone as it wasn't really the individuals I had a problem with - it was the system which was too rigid, too dehumanizing, too impersonal, too toxic, and too superior to admit it. People just didn't realize what they had chosen to believe in.

I've seen so many people die because they had to listen to their friends, relatives and doctors about what to do. They began a healing program, then asked their doctor about it. The doctor said it was a waste of time and that they were delaying urgently needed medical treatment. Next thing I knew, they died of a complication or from the poisoning of the chemotherapy. They followed the doctors because their relative had said something like, "You can't continue this healing program - you need more protein, more food!" They followed the medical treatment and died. I believe a person has to decide whether or not they want to live, and they have to stick by their decisions no matter what. It does not have to alienate everyone, but we cannot live our lives controlled by the opinions of those around us. We must take that very scary step onto center stage, ignore our fears, and shine our brilliance everywhere.

We have to dare to have an original thought, to travel on the unbeaten path, to go where we want to go. In the end, it is only our own opinion about our life that matters anyway. Ask yourself - whose opinion about how I lived my life will matter to me when I'm on my deathbed? Usually people when they're dying tell us that they wished they would have lived their life the way they wanted to, not the way everyone else wanted them to live it. They would've gone to architecture school, not business school. They would have become a scientist, not a lawyer. They would have become an artist, not a school teacher. Or they would have become a school teacher, not a doctor. Don't wait until the end of your life, when it's too late to make these decisions about what to do with your life. It really is that important.

Internal Medicine

Scut, Competition and Faulty Labs

Nothing was to prepare me for the chaos and the hard work that followed. I found out quickly that the students were turned loose into the system with hardly any idea of what was going on.

Compared to the first two years of school, there was no longer any sort of structure to what we were to study. If we wanted to learn a procedure, we were to find someone who was doing one and watch it. Then, when the opportunity came up, volunteer to do one. They called it "See one, do one, teach one" because as soon as you had seen it once, you were supposed to be able to do it, and once you had done it once, you were supposed to be able to teach someone else how to do it. Easier said than done.

We students learned to rely on each other so much. I would be walking through the hall trying to find someone to help me because a patient's veins were so hardened from old age and disease that I couldn't get any blood out of them. One patient had fatty tumors all around the arm area where one takes the blood, and I couldn't draw blood from him, either. Then, there were the patients whose veins were all collapsed because they had been in the hospital so long, and so many technicians had come before to take their blood.

Everyone I approached was busy - the nurses - giving medication, the technicians - doing paperwork, the residents - in with patients and monstrous amounts of paperwork. The attending physician - never could be found. A medical student, overloaded with his own patients, would yell out, "Use a butterfly needle." What's a butterfly needle? Then along would come another medical student who had just enough time to show me where the butterfly needles were and quickly scurried off to do what we called "scut." Then another would show up and say, "Do it like this." Still I wouldn't know what I was doing. Finally, I would just walk in the room with the patient and try the best I could. If one didn't do it that way, one could be standing there all day long, never getting anything done.

Since the students and residents are not adequately trained to do what they're doing, when patients walk into a teaching hospital, they are being worked on and experimented on. Many times the relatives of the patients were aware of this fact, and they would yell at me if I didn't get a blood draw right the first time. I had to learn patience in these circumstances. They were usually sorry afterwards, as I was always gracious. Considering the horrible lack of supervision in teaching hospitals, a medical student may be the closest person to a licensed doctor that people will ever see.

"Scut" we called it. These were the unpleasant chores that no one wanted to do, the ones that the medical students had to do because they were last on the totem pole - things like checking lab tests, retrieving X-rays, relaying messages between residents and attendings, drawing blood (technicians were supposed to do that), getting supplies for the residents, tracking down old records, retrieving information from other hospitals regarding the patient in question, taking lab tests to the lab, and anything else that none of the staff wanted to do. We all knew about scut work and were told that we were supposed to do everything we were told and have a smile on our face because our attitude was a major determinant of our grade. And so we were prepped.

Patients stayed way too long in this particular hospital because the stay was already paid for. The longer they stayed, the sicker they became, and the more likely they picked up nosocomial infections. The residents even joked about it. They said, "We had better hurry up and get so-and-so out of here before he picks up an infection. You know, the longer the patient stays in the hospital, the sicker he gets." It was not only spoken, it was true. The longer I saw them stay, the more complications they suffered, and the more they came down with infections. Then we would do the whole antibiotic vicious cycle again.

It was disheartening to learn the truth about so many things. One shock was that there were so many mistakes made with giving the proper medications. The most common was to miss a dose of something or to completely eliminate a medication from the schedule. There were lists that were kept in the nurses' rolling carts that showed what medications were given and when, and we were told to check these lists every day because it was so common for the medications not to be given correctly. What was annoying was that in order to get to the list, we had to get a key from a nurse which meant we had to *find* the nurse. I don't know where they hid. I don't know what they did, but I could rarely find them. I went searching from room to room, hoping to find them with the patients. As I looked into each room, I would hear the desperate plea again, "Have you seen my doctor? Please find my doctor. I haven't seen my doctor in over a week!" To find a doctor, *too*, this was really too much to ask!

I don't mean to discount the work of nurses. I applaud them for putting up with so much mistreatment from doctors as well as from the patients. They were the ones who had to take care of the wounds - they saw the medication side effects that were frequently so severe. They were the ones who saw up close and personal the emotional and physical devastation caused by medicine. Maybe this is one of the reasons why nurses have been at the head of the holistic health movement. They have seen firsthand what medicine does. It's so easy for doctors to prescribe and give an invasive treatment or procedure when they don't have to follow up all day long with the patient's condition minute by minute like the nurses so often do. Doctors many times have no idea how much it hurts to recover from a procedure, from a side effect, or from a surgery.

The residents taught me many things. They told me the very best medical reference text I could get was the _____ manual. It was a diagnostic and treatment manual that described the signs and symptoms of the different diseases, how to diagnose the disease or condition and how to treat it. It was easy to read, not too long, and contained plenty of information. They said, "Get the _____ manual, but don't quote from it because it's written by a drug company and that's considered biased information." Then they would tell me if I quoted that manual, to say it came from Harrison's text instead which was considered a reliable source of medical information. There were so many reference manuals out there, and doctors had so little time to read them, that they wouldn't know the difference between a quote from one book or the other.

I'll never forget the patient who came in with severe shortness of breath. He was in heart failure, and his lungs regularly filled up with fluid. In these cases, the fluid is usually drained as much as possible from the lungs and the fluid is sent to the lab to be analyzed for inflammatory conditions, uncomplicated fluid buildup (called a pleural effusion), cancer, or infection.

Since this was considered a relatively easy procedure to do, the residents allowed me to do the draining (called a thoracentesis). A thoracentesis is defined as a surgical puncture of the chest wall for the removal of fluids. I had never done one of these before, so the resident was there with me teaching me how to do it. I stuck a very large hollow needle into his back between his ribs in the lung area. The needle was attached to some tubing that led to a large, gallon-sized glass bottle on the floor. Of course it was painful for the patient. As I guided the needle in, the fluid commenced flowing out through the tubing, so we knew we had placed the needle correctly. The resident decided that she had too many things to do to just sit there and watch fluid drain out of the man's lung, so she left for a few minutes, saying she needed to catch up on some paperwork. Everything seemed to be going well.

In a couple of minutes, the man started yelling in pain and complaining that he couldn't breathe. There I was holding the needle in his back, and I couldn't let go of it to find the resident who could have been anywhere. I was stuck holding the needle, praying as hard as I could that the resident would come back. I had no idea what was wrong, and the only thing I could do was hold his hand and tell him to stay calm. He was laboring to breathe, but he seemed stable.

The resident came back in a few minutes and ordered a chest X-ray. It is routine to do the X-ray after this procedure because of the risk of collapsing a lung during a thoracentesis. It showed he had a collapsed lung. I've never felt so bad in my entire life. It was the first time that I had ever felt like I hurt someone. I didn't just inconvenience him; I caused him major suffering. Doctors like to talk about the risk vs. benefit ratio for doing a procedure. They talk about it with a dry clinical tone in their voices. If the benefit is greater than the risk, then doctors like to say that the risk is acceptable, and that justifies doing the procedure. They talk about the risk being acceptable as if it were a machine they were referring to - not a human life.

There was a surgery consult, and a surgery resident came, made a large incision in his chest and stuck a large tube through it into the lung area which would be attached to tubing which would, in turn, be attached to the wall which provided suction. The suction would create a vacuum and cause his lung to re-expand. The tube is horribly painful, as I had seen other patients who had this procedure done, and for as long as the tube stayed in, the patients usually were always screaming for more pain medication. He didn't complain, though, and this really bothered me. He seemed to be one of those stoic types who never let on how much he hurt. It only made me feel guiltier.

Granted, a collapsed lung is a risk of the thoracentesis

procedure, and it has happened many other times during this procedure, I began to fully grasp what it meant to have a "complication." I also began to understand fully the phrase - "Do no harm." Medicine and I did harm to him that day. For some reason, I was the only one upset about it. Everyone else seemed to accept it very matter-of-factly as just one of the many complications that can occur. This is because these complications were happening all the time, and they were so common that doctors didn't even get upset about them any-more. Medical techniques had become so invasive that when a patient suffered from a mishap, it was just accepted. People die at the hands of medicine; people get seriously hurt. This was not a game; this was real life. I thought I was going to medical school to help people, not hurt them!

Medicine doesn't know what else to do for a lung filled with fluid. They don't know about lobelia, or juice fast-ing, or intestinal cleansing, or the many other lung herbs out there. They don't know about cayenne, hydrotherapy, castor oil packs, etc. They had no idea how to help him except to drain the fluid out of his lungs with a large needle. Since it is so invasive, it carries certain risks. When was it ever put down as a law that when something goes wrong with the body that we have to cut inside the body and take it out? This seems to be the philosophy of modern medicine.

This patient was in the hospital for many weeks, so I remember him vividly. His name was Mr. Chagaro. We rounded on him every morning, and I also checked on him every afternoon. The resident taking care of him mispro-nounced his name every day. After a week or so, I started correcting her. She still couldn't get it. It was not a hard name to say. I don't blame her because I know how much residents are overworked, and I know she had way more patients than she could handle. But that is nothing new in medical training. She had so many patients, she couldn't remember their names. I'm surprised she remembered what was wrong with all of them.

I thought it interesting that although she couldn't pronounce his name, she could very easily pronounce the name of his affliction (exudative pleural effusion) - a far more complicated phrase to say and remember. It was very common to refer to patients by the name of their disease instead of by their name. We would hear, "Go check out the malignant liver tumor in room four," or "There's a diabetic in room one," or "The epileptic down the hall is depressed." I wanted to know their names.

If we can't get our patients' names right, how do we call ourselves doctors? Maybe we should call ourselves human scientists because we understand lab values and tests and the theories of disease. But do we understand human beings? If we are not connecting with our patients, how do we call ourselves doctor? I've heard that the word doctor comes from the Latin root which means teacher, but there was no instruction of the patient in this hospital. There was no teaching him how to heal himself, what techniques to use to make himself stronger, and how to live a healthy lifestyle to ensure this sort of thing didn't happen again. There was only an air of detached science pervading his hospital room.

I wish that were the end, but his lab values came back showing that the fluid we drained out of his lung was infected. He developed high fevers, and appeared to worsen. In addition, his blood tests showed he was anemic. While the doctors debated the cause of his anemia, he seemed to become even sicker. They pontificated about the pus pockets in his lungs. They wondered if he were bleeding from his lungs. They thought, maybe he was anemic because he was bleeding from somewhere in his intestines, and proceeded to schedule him for multiple tests to check his intestinal tract for bleeding. They sent him downstairs to swallow barium to check his upper GI tract. Then they sent him to have barium shot up his rectum to check his lower GI tract. Then they decided that they would have a look inside his colon with a colon scope (called a colonoscopy) just to be sure. They found nothing. Meanwhile, the residents were checking his blood every day to monitor the infection.

I came in early to check all the endless lab tests, many of which were inaccurate. In fact, so many times, the numbers did not make sense, and I would ask a resident, "Why is this lab value this? It doesn't make sense!" I received the standard reply, "Ignore, it - it's a lab error." I became very frustrated as I soon began to wonder which lab tests I *could* trust. The doctors' answer to this dilemma was to merely keep on repeating the blood test until they got consistent numbers among the many tests.

I used to muse at the fact that the doctors were not telling the patients that they thought the lab had messed up; they simply would state that the test needed to be repeated because the "results were inconclusive." This fancy languaging given with the right authoritative tone resulted in a passive acceptance by the patients. They had no choice, anyway. They knew they had to do what the doctor said. They were in a hospital bed hooked up to an I.V. I mean, they were a captive audience. Who's going to argue when they feel horrible, they have an IV stuck in their arm, they've just had a very painful procedure done to them, they're wearing a hospital gown that opens in all the wrong places, and they can't get any sleep because the guy next to them either snored or was watching TV all night in a different language!

With all of the errors, I found it ludicrous that doctors relied on lab values so heavily. I had been taught that a good history and physical exam were all that was needed 95% of the time in order to diagnose a disease. For some reason, we have taken lab tests to be better indicators than our own common sense and clinical judgment. I remember our professors used to tell us repeatedly, "Touch your patients." They wanted us to connect with the patients, and let them know that we cared. One of the easiest way to do that was with a reassuring touch - maybe on the shoulder. One of the reasons they had to tell us that in school was because nowadays, doctors hardly touch or even talk to their patients much anymore. They take lab tests, and use those lab tests to determine what's going on. This is why people complain that they don't feel they are being treated like a human being. It is because the humanity has been taken out of the doctor visit.

The most bothersome about the lab tests was that they were usually not performed on time. I would rush to call the lab in the morning to get the answer sooner, and they would tell me that the sample hadn't even arrived. Or, I'd go down to X-ray to check on X-rays ordered two days ago, and the X-ray had not even been taken. Eventually, It got so bad that I resorted to wheeling down the patients myself to the X-ray department and literally accompanying them through the whole process.

I didn't rely on anybody at all to do anything, and pretty soon, I was wearing about 6 different hats. I played nurse, tech, clerk, medical student, phlebotomist, and at times, resident. It was the only way anything got done. In fact, the residents used to commonly say, "If you want anything done around here, you have to do it yourself." Some resorted to writing all of their orders "STAT" - meaning urgent. That way, the test was performed in two days instead of two weeks. However, an order written STAT is supposed to be reserved for emergencies only. People moved like molasses in this hospital, and they didn't care if they got their job done now or 10 days later - they still got paid.

One day, my anemic patient told me he knew the reason for his low blood count. He very confidently announced that the reason he was anemic was because we were drawing his blood every day to do the blood tests. Smart patient. I discussed this fact with the residents (not the ones responsible for him), and discovered it was actually documented that patients can become anemic from frequent blood draws. We decided at my vehement request against checking his blood so frequently.

There was more, though. After multiple analyses of his lung fluid, he turned out to have a type of lung cancer. This man had been through multiple procedures, suffered many complications of the many procedures he had undergone, and now the residents told him they wanted to do a biopsy to see what kind of cancer it was. He flat out told them *no*, emphatically stating he was leaving the hospital. Everyone was shocked except for me. Maybe no one stopped to consider how it felt to be him.

The day of his discharge from the hospital, I walked into his room where he was lying comfortably, looking like he was already halfway recovered from the day before, solely because he was leaving the torture chamber (oops, I mean hospital). He had a wide grin on his face, and told me how happy he was to be leaving. Whoever said that if a person has cancer, they have to do all of this toxic chemotherapy that can make him violently ill, and which research studies show do not prolong his life, but will make his tumor shrink temporarily? Whatever empowers the patient, whatever lights up the patient, I have to trust is the right thing for them to do. Who said he had to do natural healing, either? Why couldn't he make his own choice? He thanked me for being the only person who was nice to him.

After several weeks, we had a new attending physician take the place of the other one. The first one had been very helpful and understanding, and she had livened up the conferences. She had been a good professor for teaching the system she was in. The second one who came on was very different. She and I started off on the wrong foot one day when she began to question our beliefs about regular mammograms.

All of the students and residents and residents assembled on a regular basis to discuss the status of the patients and what treatment plan to follow with them. Opening up a discussion about mammograms, she began with the question, "Would you personally get regular mammograms? Would you recommend mammograms for your mother? And would you recommend mammograms for your patients?" I was the only one who said I wouldn't have them ever. As soon as I had said it, I realized what I had done, and I could see every jaw in the room hit the floor. Big OOPS. Too late to take it back. I had to own what I had said.

This time, I wanted to stand my ground and tell the

truth. I was asked a direct question, and I felt it deserved a direct answer. Usually, I wasn't asked so directly, and I could skirt all the way around the issue while seeming to answer it, when in reality I had not. This time, I told the truth. I said I did not want my breasts to be exposed to radiation - something every scientist and doctor knows causes cancer. But that wasn't all. I could have stopped there, but I was on a roll. She queried, "Aren't you worried about missing a breast cancer?" I added that I felt confident that I knew the things to do to prevent cancer, and I thought because of my healthy lifestyle that I would never have to worry about cancer. (I have even more confidence in natural healing now than I did then. If one knows how to heal it, one does the same thing to prevent it - one definitely knows how to prevent it because it's the same thing as healing it.) You should have seen the eyes go wide open and the jaws go down again. She didn't bother to ask me about the details of my so-called healthy lifestyle, but continued on with the discussion. I didn't grasp the importance of what I had just said -- it was a personal issue with her, especially since she was around the age when breast cancer usually strikes.

After the discussion, she mentioned that breast cancer ran in her family. She said that she would never consider doing chemotherapy, and she had left instructions with every family member that if she was ever diagnosed with breast cancer, she didn't want any treatment except that they hook her up to a morphine drip and let her go "peacefully." It obviously was a highly charged issue for her. It would be important for her to have regular mammograms, so that the doctors could find it early. But, she really did not want to hear it that if she got breast cancer, it was because of the diet and lifestyle she had been leading. She would rather have thought that it was some unlucky fate that caused breast cancer to run in her family, and that she had no responsibility whatsoever in creating it. I was threatening something very near and dear to her - her belief in her own victimhood. How dare I!

To wrap up, she discussed the relevance of a research

study that ultimately showed that mammograms are no more effective at finding breast cancer than a breast self-exam. There are normally many research studies out there that contradict each other. You could quote a research study to support pretty much anything you wanted to say.

I had implied that she was wrong for having mammograms. No wonder she gave me a D on my evaluation. Doing the same amount of work and studying, I received an A from the first professor and a D from the second. I guess she made her feelings known to me in an indirect way - a D. From then on, I kept my mouth shut. No attending from then on had any idea I was even remotely into natural healing or even taking vitamins.

Very recently I received a call from a lady who requested the specific recipe for the herbal poultice to apply in order to regrow new tissue. I asked her why she needed the poultice, and she replied that she had been doing an herbal program, and in addition, she had been using a different poultice that drew out her baseball-sized cancer, and now there was a hole in her breast where the cancer used to be. She needed the poultice recipe in order to grow new breast tissue in its place.

She told me that at the end of 1998, the doctors told her she had one week to live, and that she had better go to a hospice to wait out her time. She was told to get her affairs in order. Her friend had shown her some information describing how to heal herself with natural healing, and she followed the directions. She simply followed the directions without knowing much of the specifics of why, and within 10 days, her tumor began to slough off in the shower. After a couple of months, she had a nurse look at it, who picked at it a bit, and the whole thing just fell off. She said it looked like a deflated balloon with long tentacles and was covered in pus, and that it was so disgusting that she almost passed out, describing the cancer in a way that only someone who had it could know. Most of us never see cancer because the doctors are always trying to cut them out. She was going to continue the cleanses until she was totally healed.

She already went through the worst part - the rest was downhill. I wanted to reach out and hug her because of her bravery. You may think she was special and I surely know that she is, but she is not rare. There are so many others who have healed themselves naturally of supposedly incurable diseases. Literally thousands have the nerve to recover in spite of being told they were going to die.

My nutritionist used these herbal poultices, and this is how she would pull out the tumors along with an herbal detoxification program for internal cleansing. It is intense healing, but that woman's breast will grow back and she will have a whole one again. Better than a mastectomy. Most importantly, she will live, and she may live for twenty or more years longer if she continues to live a healthy lifestyle.

I have been introduced to a few other centers in the United States where people go who have been told they had something incurable. I have been to some of them personally. Many afflicted with different cancers - pancreatic, leukemia, breast cancer, melanoma, liver cancer, colon cancer, brain cancer, and other diseases such as multiple sclerosis, lupus, and other diseases too numerous to list, come to these centers after the cancer has already spread to the bones and everywhere else, and they've been told by their doctors to go home and die. At the centers, they fill up these patients with fresh juices, sprouts and wheatgrass juice, and have them do a lot of intestinal cleansing. The patients heal themselves of their so-called "incurable" diseases.

Incurable is a state of mind. Hope, faith and belief move mountains. They compel people to do something about their predicament. People who believe the lie that they are incurable will hear of a natural healing program, but because they truly believe they cannot be healed, they will only try halfway. They only heal halfway, and then they die. When they believe in the possibility, they decide to do everything possible to help themselves - they are asking the question, "What else can I do to heal myself?" Not surprisingly, they get great results – *not* spontaneous remissions. These people work very hard to change their lifestyles and to eat only fresh, chemical-free food and to cleanse the old, accumulated filth and toxins out of their body that caused the cancer in the first place.

But, we did not get such great results at the hospital. I learned many other things during our morning discussions/rounds. One day, we discussed coronary heart disease and the treatment available for it. When a patient came in with angina pains, and the angiogram showed his (usually *his*) coronary arteries were clogged up with cholesterol, there were a few options available. One was to have a coronary bypass surgery that I've already discussed. Even doctors know how dangerous and invasive this surgery can be, which is why there was another technique developed called angioplasty which was considered less invasive.

During an angioplasty (means surgery on blood vessels), a tube is inserted through the major leg vein and threaded up through the heart to the coronary blood vessels which are clogged. Then an instrument is used, either an inflatable balloon which, when inflated, squashes the cholesterol against the sides of the blood vessel walls, making the opening wider, or an instrument which scrapes the cholesterol off the walls. Both were associated with a 60% chance of the blood vessels closing off again in the next 6 months to 2 years. It was said that this is because these instruments damage the lining of the blood vessels during this process, and that the arteries close off not with cholesterol, but with scar tissue due to the trauma of the procedure. But these procedures were preferred to the coronary bypass surgery because the risks of infection, dying, and pneumonia were so much less. The only problem was that in 6 months to a few years when the blood vessels closed off with scar tissue, everyone would need the coronary bypass surgery anyway.

With all of these sick patients around me, I still had to go home and deal with my own sick self. Some days during my own healing, I would cry to Claire that I didn't think I could continue. I had too much pain, it was too hard, and I just couldn't do it anymore. I was trying to keep up a grueling third year medical student's schedule while at the same time doing a full-time healing program, and I still was very weak. I was still lying on the floor many hours out of the day, and still in pain, although not as much. There were times I lost hope and just *knew* I couldn't.

She would grab my arm with such intensity, look me straight in the eyes with her eyes penetrating mine and she would say emphatically, "Yes, you can! You are *already* doing it." She would say it with such unwavering faith that I believed her. I got back to working hard on my healing. She had such a persuasive way about her. One of the most powerful things about her was the way she was able to reach out and affect people - profoundly. No medical doctor had ever affected me in that way. No ordinary medical doctor knows how much courage and persistence it takes to fight a deadly disease and win.

In the hospital, I saw my first patient with acalculous cholecystitis. The layman's term for this would be a gallbladder attack, but without the gallstones. A gallbladder attack is mostly due to the presence of stones in the gallbladder; however, sometimes it is caused by the fluid bile in the gallbladder getting too thick, "sludging" in the gallbladder which caused irritation and pain. The treatment for it was removal of the gallbladder. The professors said it was common for it to happen to people who had been in the hospital for long periods of time and who had taken many medications. Since I knew that most drugs must be processed and detoxified in the liver from 2nd year pharmacology, I knew it was from the long-term exposure to all of those chemicals in the drugs. Being in the hospital and taking multiple medications was the only cause of acalculous cholecystitis.

Because so many medical students were working so diligently to display such a great attitude and to do more than what was expected for a grade, there was sometimes intense competition between students. I never ran into a problem until I hit Internal Medicine. As I mentioned before, we joked about certain students, calling them "Gunners," because they were off and going as soon as the gun went off, so to speak. They were always doing more, staying later, quoting obscure articles in nauseating and even irrelevant detail - *especially* irrelevant details.

The gunner's name was Stewart. For me to do only what was required made me look like a D student next to him, so I began to come in earlier just to keep up with him. As I came up the hospital elevator one morning, a doctor asked me what was I doing there so early, and I told him the story of Stewart the Gunner. He empathized with words that know. We've all been there.

Stewart began to do things to sabotage me and make me look bad. I remember there was an internal medicine outpatient clinic we were supposed to go to on Wednesday afternoons. He told me the clinic got canceled. Imagine my surprise when the resident asked me if I was going to the clinic, and I answered, "It was canceled." The resident replied, "No, it's not - who told you that?" Imagine my further surprise when I got to the outpatient clinic and who showed up but my favorite gunner - Stewart!

From then on, whenever he told me something, I always confirmed it with someone else. I also told my attending about it. We talk about how doctors are supposed to have such a highly developed sense of ethics. I wasn't going to let someone get through medical school getting away with sabotaging others (He got through anyway, and so did the many others). Medicine encourages that fierce competition between students so that they cheat and sabotage each other.

I thought it was a rare occurrence that something like that happened to me, but when I talked to my friends about it on other rotations, they **all** had stories to tell me about how such-and-such tried to sabotage them and make them look bad. The reasoning was if you make someone else look bad, you thus make yourself look good and land yourself a good grade.

One of Stewart's patients was a brittle diabetic who

was admitted to the hospital to have his insulin dose adjusted. A brittle diabetic is one whose diabetes is very difficult to control. Mr. Needel was a very bitter man, and none of the staff liked to be around him because he was always full of complaints. He wouldn't follow the recommended diabetic diet in the hospital, so he just ate what he wanted. But if you were told that your diabetes was incurable, and that you could control it with insulin, wouldn't you just eat whatever you wanted, too? I mean, life is short -- why shouldn't we just eat whatever pleases us?

Diabetics are at increased risk for getting infections because their immune systems are not very strong, and their high blood sugar is a very rich source of nutrients for all sorts of microorganisms. Since the hospital is the best place to pick up an infection, one day he developed an infection that would keep him in the hospital for months. He had been admitted solely for a few days of adjusting his insulin dose. The resident noticed that the man's knee was red and hot and diagnosed a joint infection. The attending wanted to treat it conservatively with antibiotics, as opposed to doing a surgery to clean out the joint. According to the research, this should have worked, but it didn't. It wasn't the first time that the flat lifeless research correlated very poorly with the actual live results we saw in the hospital. I frequently wondered who was doing all of this research that it supported the use of drugs which did not appear to work, even though the research stated that they did. Something was not right about it.

A surgery consult was called in, and as the surgeon was examining the patient for the first time in our presence, he took the opportunity to tell us that we should have called him right away, and that the attending had made the wrong decision to treat him with antibiotics only. He quoted some obscure research study, proving his point that an infected joint should be immediately surgically cleaned out. He took several jabs at the attending about how she had done the wrong thing, and the next thing I knew, everyone was looking up research studies trying to support the decision they had made. It was the hot debate. It was something we called a "turf battle," meaning that the doctors were fighting over who should care for the patient - internal medicine or surgery? They each thought Mr. Needel should be on their "turf". Either of them could have been right depending on which research study you decided to believe.

The surgeons cleaned out his joint and created even worse problems. He emerged from surgery with a huge gash all down the side of his thigh from the surgery. Since doctors know wounds heal very badly in a brittle diabetic, surgery can be *very* risky in this case. Well, his wound would *not* heal. Since the research studies showed that using a whirlpool could help wounds heal faster, the doctors decided to send him to the whirlpool and for hyperbaric oxygen a couple of times per week. However, the patient then developed a particular bacterial infection called pseudomonas. Well, the research studies also stated that one can pick up pseudomonas infections from whirlpools because that particular bacteria thrives in the hot temperatures there. The dreaded pseudomonas caused a greenish material to be exuded from the wound and further delayed its healing. We checked on the green wound every day. It did not improve.

I did notice something interesting about doctors at that point. We were all gathered around looking at the green wound, and everyone was disgusted but trying not to show it. Doctors are always hiding their true feelings, and in many cases, this is desirable depending on the situation. But I learned how a doctor deals with these unpleasant feelings is by intellectualizing them. That is, if a doctor can spout off a lot of theories and research about the pseudomonas infection and the particular details about the treatment, it makes the doctor forget about the disgusting green wound, and makes him feel more comfortable. Doing this makes the doctor more in control - he's in control of his own knowledge while the fear is that he is not in control of the wound. He has no idea what's going to happen to the patient, and this is the utter truth.

I think hearing the details sometimes helps the patients, too, because they can name the enemy - it's pseudomonas, and we're going to fight this enemy with A, B, and C methods and drugs. They are comforted by this, unless they develop a complex about why their doctor won't tell them in plain English what is wrong with them.

The professors during our first two years of school taught us to always attempt to explain medicine to patients in language they could understand. During the third and fourth years, that teaching went right out the window. Either the doctor didn't have time to translate to English in his own mind, or the doctor actually wanted to keep an advantage over the patient by keeping them ignorant so they would be more likely to follow his advice later.

I took special time to explain terms to my patients. When I asked them, "Do you know what _____ means? This is the procedure/ drug you are about to take. Do you know what _____ means? This is the name of your disease." They always replied that they had no idea what it was. Sometimes these patients had had a particular disease for years, and they still didn't know what it meant! I had so much educating to do. Educating took time, however, and I was always at the hospital, and always being at the hospital exhausted me. I did the best I could. Someone had to tell them. Someone had to teach them.

Meanwhile, Stewart was very diligent about keeping those blood sugars in the normal range the whole time, but it didn't make any difference at all in the patient's condition.

You can't heal a person by trying to keep a number in the "normal" range. What's going on with a person is so much bigger than just a number. Blood sugar was only the beginning of what was wrong with him. His liver was clogged up with environmental toxins and medications, his attitude was horrible, his diet was deplorable, and definitely not health-building, his colon was filthy and overloaded with years of putrefied waste. No wonder his immune system wouldn't work. And no one ever addressed his subconscious death wish.

Finally, our group of students went on to our next rotation, and the diabetic went to intensive care. I heard about his death a few weeks later. He got his wish. The internist and surgeons argued over whose fault is was **("...if you had only done this, if you had only done this differently, if you hadn't done that...")**. It was like watching vultures fight each other over a dead piece of carcass.

Speaking of deadly infections, there was one that was the most feared: Vanc-resistant enterococcus. This was a particular strain of enterococcus (intestinal bacteria) that had developed resistance to all antibiotics including the very powerful, but highly toxic one of last resort. A patient on the floor developed this infection, requiring risk management to be notified. The lady from risk management was barking out endless orders, and the patient was put in isolation. Every inch of the room was sterilized. There were elaborate decontamination procedures to be followed. It was important because it was known that this kind of infection could spread like wildfire through hospitals.

People were in the hospital because they were sick with something. There were huge numbers of people with weakened immune systems in the hospital - the elderly, infants, AIDS patients, cancer patients, patients undergoing chemotherapy and radiation, people eating the hospital food, people on steroids and immune suppressant drugs - the people with organ transplants, lupus, autoimmune disorders, people on kidney dialysis, etc. (Seems like almost every drug or procedure in the hospital weakened the immune systems) This is one of the reasons why it was so easy to get an infection in the hospital. It never made sense to me why they ever decided to put sick people all together in the same place so they could infect each other.

I wondered why they did not just give him charcoal that would have absorbed the infection and he would have been done with it in two days. They knew about the power of charcoal to absorb medication from the intestines when a person came in to the emergency room with a drug overdose, but somehow they had overlooked charcoal's ability to absorb bacteria and bacterial toxins from the intestines, too. In fact, charcoal has been used this way for centuries and is very effective.

The next patient came in a coma because he had had congestive heart failure for so long. So, the blood from his heart had backed up and engorged his liver because his heart couldn't pump it around his body, and it severely damaged his liver. He had the same symptom as an alcoholic with liver failure from cirrhosis - coma. Of course, his heart failure had been managed with medications. He had previously been told that they could **control** his condition, but not that he could ever be healed from it.

Congestive heart failure is usually the result of having coronary artery disease with repeated heart attacks that damage the heart or from long-standing high blood pressure that overstrains the heart for years until it finally gives out. Depending on which side of the heart is affected, the left or the right, the blood backs up into the lungs or the liver and other abdominal organs. The doctors had never heard of the thousands of people all over the world who had healed their hearts with cayenne pepper. He might have been healed years ago, and he might never have showed up in the hospital now. But the doctors still thought it was controversial to treat high cholesterol with niacin - a B vitamin, even though it was cheaper with less side effects than any other medication out there. Cayenne would have been out of the question. It was hot. People might complain.

Another patient, Mr. Smith, was admitted with a serious lung disease called pulmonary fibrosis, which is a condition in which the lungs gradually scar up over the years until the person can no longer breathe and suffocates to death. The scar tissue is stiff and does not expand like lung tissue, so the person cannot expand his lungs with air. According to the research studies, the resident should have given him a particular antibiotic combined with a steroid. The next morning after he received the recommended treatment, I walked into his room and tried to wake him up. The nurse told me he wasn't

breathing. I barely felt a pulse. Because he had a Do Not Re-
suscitate order in his chart, he was to be allowed to die with
no extraordinary measures to save him like CPR, adrenaline,
the heart defibrillator, etc. I stood there waiting for him to
wake up, still feeling his feeble pulse which eventually
stopped. Gradually, his arm turned cold in my hand, and I,
not wanting him to be dead, kept yelling in his ear to wake up.
He never woke up. It was the first time I ever saw someone
die, and it shocked me horribly. I had no idea what to do, but
somehow I knew that there should be some sort of dignified
way that he should leave his body.

The nurse couldn't understand why I was still there.
She said something like, "He's dead, so what? I've got work
to do." People die in hospitals all the time. I guess it doesn't
make an impression anymore. But since medicine teaches all
of its staff to treat bodies so invasively with surgeries, drugs
and radiation, they become just that - inanimate, anonymous
bodies with a particular name of a disease but with no personal identity or humanity. So when they die - so what? I
wished him well, and prayed for him that he would make it
safely to his next destination. It felt strange to be praying over
a dead body, but I knew he had an identity, and I knew there
was something else to being a human being, I knew that
something survives after death.

The worst part about the hospital was not necessarily
the death I saw. I know none of us like to face the fact that
we're going to die someday. I like to think about how I have
so many years ahead of me - that I can do anything I want to
do with my life, and that I have unlimited time. I don't like to
think about the fact that it will end one day. I saw it end for
so many people. I didn't want it to end for them. I didn't
want them to die with regrets.

I didn't want them to die with bitterness the way I
knew I would have died if I hadn't gone to see Claire that first
day. I knew how much it hurt to feel as if I were dying and to
know the agony and the despair that I hadn't lived my life
fully, that I had not tried something new because I just knew

I wasn't good enough, that I hadn't spoken up for myself when people treated me badly, and that I didn't ask the handsome man out because I was too shy and felt too badly about myself. I didn't have my life all figured out when I thought I was going to die. I didn't want this to happen to all of these dying people. I wanted them to have extra time - at least to say their truth, to speak their mind, to live the way they would have lived if they had only known that they had such a short time before they would be told that horrible truth, "You're going to die," when they weren't ready to hear it.

If we could only have it our way. If we only knew when we were going to die. Maybe then we would know how well or how badly to treat our bodies. If we only knew when it was God's time to say, "You've lived all that you're supposed to live, and you're going to have to leave now." But we don't know that at all. We can't possibly know what's around the corner. All we can do is hope that we live now every way that we possibly want to live and to love ourselves as much as we can, taking the best care of our bodies that we know how to do. All we can do is try to love each other the most we can and forgive each other when we mess up. I would risk my entire career to help them all because now I understand the meaning of love.

Hospital Nutrition

The SAD Truth

The class was called "Therapeutic Nutrition." It was conducted in a private room in the hospital cafeteria. We studied eight different diets. Each time, there were lectures on a different therapeutic diet that was also accompanied by a sample meal of the diet we were studying.

I already knew it was going to be a problem. The meals were merely variations on the Standard American Diet that was highly processed, full of refined sugar, saturated fat and cholesterol and little fiber. The Standard American Diet has been referred to by many nutritionists, healers, and health educators as the SAD diet because the results of eating it did turn out to be sad. There was nothing magical or healing about these diets. They were still full of the same processed foods. Non-dairy low fat whipped cream - it's full of at least 20 different chemicals. I mean, what is in that stuff, anyway; does anyone really know? How could we possibly think that it could be therapeutic to put that in our bodies? They should have called it a maintenance diet - a diet to maintain you at the same level of sickness that you're already at now, if not make you a little worse. The categories were Low Calorie Diet For Obesity, Low Protein/ Liver Failure Diet, Low Potassium Diet for kidney failure, Lactose Free Diet, Low Sodium Diet for high blood pressure, Low Cholesterol Diet, and the Hypoglycemic Diet. After I had been making and eating my own fresh food for several months now, to eat this processed food tasted like lifeless cardboard. I could literally taste the chemicals. I understood why and how so many patients in the hospital kept worsening and couldn't seem to recover from their illnesses and surgery. With the horrible hospital diet, they didn't have a chance. They were not getting enough nutrients, vitamins, minerals, etc. in order to build new tissue to heal up their surgical wounds.

I had already anticipated a problem with my eating the meals, so I telephoned the nutrition professor, Dr. Staup, to let her know I would have special dietary requirements. Her official title was Professor for the Division of Gastroenterology and Nutrition in the Department of Nutrition. I figured with a title like that, she would be very knowledgeable about different kinds of nutrition programs. Evidently, she had never heard of the unprocessed, unrefined real food diet that heals people. Of course, she inquired why I required special arrangements, and I tried to be as vague as possible, but she was one of those professors trying to rescue me from the clutches of fraudulent quackery again.

I told her I was seeing a nutritionist in town, and she asked who it was. When I told her, she literally screamed, "You'd better not follow any of that woman's advice, and you'd better not take anything she tells you to take. I know her! She's a quack! She's not even a licensed dietitian!" It sounded like the basis of her judgment of Claire as a quack rested solely on the fact that Claire was not a licensed dietitian. I thought, Oh boy, I've been following her advice for months now and I'm healthier - it's a little too late to turn back now. I just shut my mouth - I didn't say anything. I just let this woman rant on the phone for a while and then I said goodbye. She needed to rant and rave for a while. Obviously something had happened in the past that had really upset her about this lady. It was so sad what she missed out on because she only looked at peoples' "official credentials." She only considered official paper certificates - empty paper awards. I suppose she thought she won the argument over the phone because she didn't bring it up with me again during class. Fine with me - pick on someone else - I'm just trying to heal myself here, and get my degree.

We learned about the Recommended Daily Allowances (the RDA) and how they were the bare minimum of the nutrients required to prevent blatant deficiency diseases like scurvy (vitamin C deficiency) and pellagra (thiamine - a B vitamin deficiency). People need much more than what the RDA is for any water-soluble nutrient in order to be healthy.

Caffeinated tea and refined sugar, and worse, artificial sweeteners, were all served with each meal. At least they served fresh lemon with the tea. That lemon wedge was the only healthy thing on the plate. Margarine with its hydrogenated trans fatty acids, which the body recognizes as foreign, was also freely available (and everyone ate it except me). Maybe they could have taken a hint from the Italians and just used olive oil and herbs with their bread. The Italians definitely have less disease than we do.

The **hypoglycemic** diet contained, among other things, buttered mashed potatoes. The mashed potatoes were made from processed, highly salted flakes to which was added water. We could see some of the undissolved flakes. The flakes had to have been so thoroughly heated that no nutrients were left in them.

The **lactose-free** diet contained that nondairy whipped topping over canned peaches with the nutrients cooked out of them and soaking in sugary syrup that didn't even taste like peaches to me. I wonder why they didn't just put a fresh peach on the plate. There was also a white bleached refined flour dinner roll, which looked like it should have just been thrown in the trash. I wouldn't even have it on my plate. They might well have called it allergy-causing, mucous-forming, acid-forming colon glue because that's what refined food does in the body.

The **low protein** diet contained a fried chicken leg. Chicken is **high** in protein. I never understood that one. FRIED?! I couldn't believe they were serving something so obviously unhealthy. Doctors are not the only ones who know that fried foods are harmful.

The **low cholesterol** diet contained - guess what - meat! Turkey to be exact. It's this low cholesterol diet with meat in it that bothers me because I've never seen it work. Every patient who I saw who tried this meat-containing diet had to be put on the cholesterol-lowering medication. Most of the cholesterol-lowering medication damaged the liver, so the patient had to keep coming back into the doctor's office regularly in order to have blood tests done to check for liver damage. Since it's the liver's job to make and to process cholesterol, damage to the liver further impairs its ability to clear out the cholesterol in the bloodstream. This means over time, the cholesterol problem will get worse while taking these medications. Would I choose liver damage or a change in my diet? I know which one I would choose.

People could eat as many fruits, vegetables, nuts, seeds, grains and tofu that they wanted and they would be eating zero cholesterol. What they would find is that in one to two months, a high cholesterol reading would return to normal.

The **low sodium** diet was prescribed for high blood pressure. It contained ground beef - something nowadays that is full of growth hormones, antibiotics, saturated fat and cholesterol and is also high in sodium. Then, there is the risk of Mad Cow Disease with eating cows in the first place. Researchers have linked the eating of red meat to a higher risk for colon and prostate cancer. But I guess that has nothing to do with high blood pressure. What do I know? I couldn't figure that one either. I thought *are they sure this is therapeutic nutrition? Maybe I got the wrong class.*

And last, but not least, the **low calorie** diet for obesity contained meat (does saturated fat help you lose weight?) and, again, those hard white flour rolls. No wonder people have such a hard time losing weight when they follow this kind of diet. The nutrients are so cooked out, so processed, so gone, that their bodies are literally starving, and thus, they cannot stop eating, even when they are full. Literally thousands of people have lost large amounts of weight by going to a vegetarian diet with an emphasis on fresh raw foods. It's not even difficult. There is no starvation. What's different about this kind of diet is that there are actually nutrients still left in it. They are healing, health-building food choices.

Later, after the series of nutrition classes was over, I heard Dr. Staup had suffered a stroke. Strokes are caused by the kind of diet people follow. Doctors know the kind of stroke she had was caused by a diet full of fat and cholesterol followed over many years. The cholesterol builds up in the arteries, and a blood clot forms on top of the cholesterol, breaks off and flies into the blood vessels of the brain where it lodges. Whatever area of the brain is nourished by that blood vessel dies, and this is a stroke.

Dr. Staup had certain beliefs about what people should eat. They were standard medical beliefs, supported by the scientific literature and research. These beliefs killed people through ignorance. Since she was living what she was teaching, at least she wasn't a hypocrite. I realized that she had been instructing doctors for years how to teach their patients how to eat so that they would end up with strokes, too. The Standard American Diet is exactly what leads to strokes. Maybe she would have fared better with the quack.

I felt so sorry for her. She had spent her whole life, dedicating it to what she thought was helping others, and it was slowly killing them. All of those days, all of those hours of work to help them, and the hours of preparation. Her overprotection of me came out of her wanting to help. You don't know how badly I just wanted to tell her the truth, not just to help her, but to help the ones she taught, to help all of the thousands in the country who need help.

I kept looking repeatedly at the doctors, their wasted efforts, the wasted time, the wasted thoughts - and instead of being angry about them not getting the fact that natural healing could save these thousands of lives that were being lost, I was so very sad. Some of them I knew wanted to be good doctors. They had studied so many years, sacrificing so many things in their lives to pursue medicine. Many of them lost their marriages because the practice of medicine was so time-consuming as well as emotionally consuming that there was no time to be an understanding, giving, emotionally available spouse. I remember the countless hours I spent on the floor studying when I couldn't stand up. I would have done anything to understand this big mystery of why people get so sick and suffer so much.

I read whole books that no one else read, but some were reading just as much as I was. They wanted to know, too. They wanted to know how to fix it and make it all better. We all just wanted to put an easy band-aid on their wounds and have them be fixed just like that. It's too scary to think we have no control over life and death. But the truth is that we have absolutely no control at all. We cannot stop death if it is time. Even in natural healing, we can stop disease, but if it is someone's destined time to die, he will be healed of his disease, and then he will die anyway for unknown reasons. God said it was time to go.

Death was a big enough issue to deal with, but the suffering - that was something else entirely. I would turn around some days and see patients left in the hallways that I swear were dead. There was so much life sucked out of them that their faces were all caved in, their eyeballs were sunken into their eye sockets, and their skin was like paper, it was so thin and dry. You could almost see the insides of them because there was no fat or muscle anymore. They would moan, and I knew the reason they were moaning was because they were too weak to yell. I remember when I was too weak to yell.

I saw so many diabetics in this hospital. It seemed everywhere I looked there was another one without any legs because they had been amputated due to poor circulation caused by the diabetes. I tortured myself with "if only's" - If only years ago, they would have tried the natural way first. If only they knew about raw foods and garlic and cayenne and hydrotherapy and more. If only they had been told they could be healed - if only I could speak the truth to them.

Maybe I am a coward. Maybe I should have spoken the truth to my professors, but I didn't. By this time, I was at the end of my third year and I really just wanted to finish medical school, so I learned to be as unobtrusive as possible. In fact, I learned how to blend in so well that I got some of my highest grades in Internal Medicine. I got glowing reports from all of my professors (except for the one with breast cancer in her family, and her evaluation didn't count for much). I was able to think more clearly, so that I could really study again, so on the Board exam in medicine, I made the highest grade, and I got a glowing recommendation from the department of Internal Medicine. They had no idea what a miracle that was. I was alive.

The biggest truth I realized was that you cannot help someone who doesn't want to be helped. You cannot heal a person. A person can be guided along the right path, but only that person knows the path. Only that person knows their life that intimately to know what is wrong with it that there is a disease. People who receive a healing heal themselves. They take the initiative and track down sources of information. They read about what can be done. They don't consider failure as an option. They experiment and try things, and then they try more things. They believe that they will find a way, and they do. Ask for what you want. If people do not want to be healed, they can go to every doctor and even every natural healer, and no one will be able to help them. They must help themselves. They are the most important doctors to themselves.

There is no such healing from a shot. There is no healing from a pill or a vaccine. There is only the healing that a person asks for, rather demands from his life. When that demand is made, a person is healed. I've dragged many a person through a natural healing routine only to realize that they didn't really want to live anyway. They wanted to stay stuck in their old patterns, too afraid to make changes. I've given some of my most brilliant inspirational speeches to people who were facing a life-threatening disease, and they said, "Yes! I've got it!" But they didn't get it, and because of that, they stopped trying and they died.

The Fourth Year

The Downward Coast

They called the fourth year the easiest year - the downward coast. There were eight weeks vacation you could take at any time during which students usually either traveled or went on interviews for residencies. Many students in my class went to Mexico or the Caribbean or Europe, but I stayed home to heal myself further.

The fourth year was still difficult for me. By this time, it looked like I was going to make it through medical school, but I had no idea what I was going to do afterwards. No one understood me.

I had learned so much about natural healing. By the time I graduated medical school, I had accumulated more natural healing books than I had medical books. I had learned that there was no such thing as an incurable disease. I had seen brain tumors healed. I had seen other cancers, migraines, hepatitis and other liver problems, lupus, and heart disease healed. I knew of many other diseases healed: bone cancer, Lou Gehrig's disease, multiple sclerosis, infertility, thyroid problems, seizures (my own and others), and many more diseases considered by the medical profession to be incurable.

I always knew that I would be healed with natural healing. I knew it from the first natural healing book I ever read. That's why when the medical doctors offered an EEG and a CAT scan to discover the cause of the seizures, I turned them down. I didn't care what particular detail caused the seizures. These things didn't matter in natural healing. I didn't want to get my mind all twisted up in an argument over this particular therapy vs. that particular therapy for this particular disease. I didn't want to read the contradictory medical opinions - and there were so many of them. I stopped reading about disturbing "diagnoses" and I put my mind on higher things: healing, love, and forgiveness. The diagnosis didn't matter. People did.

C H A P T E R   20

Radiology

Not A Pretty Picture

With that attitude, I began the first rotation of the
fourth year. As I had wanted to be a radiologist, I was very
happy to finally be taking a radiology rotation. It soon became
apparent, though, that it wasn't what I expected. First of all,
radiologists didn't just look at X-rays and read them. They
had expanded their duties to include things such as inserting
catheters into the body to drain pus out using radiologically-
guided instruments. They were almost like surgeons in this
respect.

Also, I began to learn about how toxic the radioactive
and iodinated dyes were that were used in order to enhance
the X-rays and CAT scans. I learned that about ½ % of all
people who received these dyes had fatal allergic reactions to
them and died. They died before they ever received a diagnosis.

There was a radioactive iodine that was used to kill
thyroids which were overactive. Since the thyroid is pretty
much the only organ that uses iodine, the radioactive iodine
when ingested, goes right to it. Since it was radioactive, it
killed wherever it went. Radioactivity as we all know, causes
cancer. But the worst part is that it totally destroyed the thyroid, so that afterwards, the patient suffered from an *underactive*
thyroid (there is hardly any of it left alive to make its own hormone), and needed to take the synthetic thyroid hormone
every day for the rest of his life. Worse, the thyroid is really

not the only organ that uses iodine - there are other organs, like the ovaries, that also use iodine in small amounts. So, the iodine was not as targeted and as specific a treatment as the doctors led us to believe. I couldn't imagine allowing a doctor to put cancer-causing radioactive material in my body and which damages more than the organ it's supposed to.

We were taught that finding a breast cancer early through regular mammograms does not increase a woman's survival time - it does not give her any more time left to live to be diagnosed earlier than later. That was a shock, but then, I already knew that from Internal Medicine. I listened to a female radiologist who specialized in reading mammograms, and she told us that women live the same amount of time whether or not they have any treatment for the breast cancer. I thought to myself - well, then, what is the point of her job? Does she realize what she has just said?

We read many X-rays, mostly chest X-rays. What was peculiar about the chest X-rays is that about half the time, the radiologist would point to the X-ray around the colon area, part of which could be seen at the bottom. He would point to multiple white round areas and ask the medical students what they were. It was a favorite "pimping" question. The answer was that sometime in the past - maybe 6 months to a year ago, the patient had received a barium swallowing test or a barium enema. Since the barium shows up white on an X-ray, this is beneficial because the doctors can see the outlines of the colon and see if there is any disease there. The only problem is now that so many people - even young ones, have diverticulosis of the intestines. Diverticulosis is caused by long-standing constipation and most of the time is asymptomatic (meaning that there are no symptoms). The barium would lodge in these pockets of weakened and bulging out intestines, and this would be visible on X-rays of the chest and of the abdomen months later. The doctors, I'm sure, told the patient that all of the barium would come out and that the barium test was routine. What I saw was that it was routine for it to lodge in the intestines for several months, maybe even years after the test.

This tells you how long things can stay stuck in the intestines. It shows you how toxic the average person's intestines are - very.

The average person is literally rotting from the inside out. He is drowning in his own waste. For some reason, we think that if we just add a chemical into our bodies that that will take care of the problems creating by our being living cesspools. Scientists in a laboratory will take the time to grow microorganisms in a nutrient broth, taking care to change the broth every day because of the waste the organism produces every day. If the broth is not changed regularly, the microorganism drowns in its own waste and dies. For some reason, we think we can be backed up in our waste and not suffer any consequences?

The first time I put a patient on an herbal intestinal cleanse, she called and said she was having white bowel movements. I thought, this is horrible; she's developed hepatitis - very few things cause white bowel movements. Then I realized, when she told me she had had a barium enema test a few months ago, that this was the rest of the barium coming out with the cleanse. I thought maybe this was a fluke until it kept happening repeatedly when more people did the intestinal cleansing.

In radiology, we learned the accuracy of X-rays. We were taught that about 75% of bone mass had to be gone before it became visible on the X-ray, which meant that the only definitive abnormality to show up on an X-ray was a bone fracture. I saw the common arthritis in peoples' spines, since it was noted in almost every X-ray. A good radiologist always noticed it, even if a back problem was not the reason why the X-ray was ordered. The subtleties of recognizing masses in the lungs had to be learned. A round mass in the lung could just be scar tissue, or it could be a fungal infection or it could be a cancer or any number of things. Mistakes were made all the time. X-rays were thrown up on the boards to show how they had been read wrong the first time, and these were used as teaching cases.

Bone scans were more sensitive. A bone scan showed the density of bone more accurately. They were used commonly as one of the ways to determine if a cancer had spread into the bones. The only problem was that the increase in bone density could be not only from cancer, but merely from arthritis or any other inflammation, or even from just being a young child who bones were still growing rapidly. It was not even considered a definitive test had to be supplemented with other tests. I didn't understand why they used it.

I kept hearing the radiologists read the scans saying that they were inconclusive. None of the tests meant anything by themselves; but if one gathered a preponderance of evidence with lab tests and X-rays and CAT scans and MRI's, one could finally make a diagnosis. All this combined with talking to the patient for probably a total of twenty minutes. No radiologist wanted to go out on a limb and say, "This is what the diagnosis is. If they were wrong, they could be sued. No one made a commitment that way. The X-rays would return with a reading like, "These findings are *suggestive* of.....but it also could be......these five other tests are recommended in order to confirm the diagnosis." When the doctors would read these to the patients, the patients would just be confused. They would ask, "Well, do I have it or not?" Then, they would be caught on that vicious diagnosis cycle on which laboratory tests are repeated until someone can make up their mind about what the patient has.

As I was passing through a particular reading area, I heard some radiologists discussing a case of a lady in her 50's with a long history of manic depression. They were talking about how ironic it was that all these years, she had a tumor growing in the temporal lobe of her brain that was mimicking the manic depression. The only reason they found it was because she couldn't take the headaches anymore - they became more and more severe, prompting a CAT scan. It must have been easy all those years to consider her as the same diagnosis. That way, she fit into a nice, neat little box which would make us all feel secure to know that nothing changes. We wouldn't have to actually talk deeply with her to wait for some gold nugget she would inadvertently utter that would be the key to the whole illness. No one ever bothered to check out her brain because she was obviously manic depressive and mental conditions hardly ever have physical components to them according to medical doctors. It's taught that for years preceding pancreatic cancer and other types of cancer, there can be a long period of depression. The cancer is probably already there during the depression, just not big enough to be detected yet with modern methods.

I wish doctors knew how many times I sat and talked with a patient for so long that they finally said something relevant about why they were sick - whether it was the relationship they were in, a previous illness they had that they forgot to mention earlier, the repainting of their house, or the loss of a job, etc. Why they were sick had nothing to do with their CAT scans. It had to do with their lives.

If only people knew to do something natural right then when the depression or anxiety or other emotional problem came on, these full-blown diseases would never develop. Depression is not just a deficiency of neurotransmitters like serotonin; it can be a sign of serious illness. The colon and liver are sluggish, the circulation to the head is sluggish and full of fat and cholesterol. The foods eaten are so processed that the lack of nutrients causes not enough neurotransmitters to be produced in the brain. The nerve cells cannot make them when they don't have the raw materials from food. As white refined sugar is considered by many to be a drug, its concentrated nature easily produces a blood sugar high that could easily be interpreted as "mania." For that matter, so do coffee and tea and other caffeinated products. As time goes on, the system further weakens until the immune system fails, the liver is completely full of thickened bile and chemicals and heavy metals. Now, serious disease can set in. The body's defenses have finally been broken down. Depression is not caused by a lack of antidepressants. When are we going to realize that there is no synthetic chemical out there that we lack that causes disease?

What would have happened if that lady had tried natural healing instead at the time she first began having the symptoms of manic depression? It wouldn't have mattered what the particular diagnosis was. By supporting the entire body, her body in its wisdom would have taken care of whatever toxicity inside that was causing the problem. In natural healing, it is less important what the particular diagnosis is, but the main thing is to concentrate on the body's inner voice and the symptoms, and these will tell you how the person is doing, how sick they are, and how much detoxification to do. If you take away the symptoms with drugs, you have no "monitor" to figure out how close you are to healing the problem. How do you know if you're healed if your only sign of the problem has been drugged into submission – temporarily. There's a reason why they are there. Symptoms are the body's early warning signs. They're there to help us if we will only listen to them instead of trying to destroy them.

Emergency Medicine

Can Anybody Find My Doctor?

We worked random day or night shifts of twelve hours each, so it was difficult to find a sleeping pattern. One day I'd be working the day shift, and the next day, I'd be working the night. A day and a half later, I'd be working the day again. I was so exhausted, and my sleep schedule so horrible that I started having more seizures. I kept dislocating my shoulder so many times that I began to experience very intense pain there, and one night, I almost agreed to have it X-rayed. I remember thinking how ridiculous it was to overwork medical students this way, only the residents had it worse: they worked 24-hour shifts. I couldn't even begin to imagine. Everyone walked around with sugar-filled snacks and multiple cups of coffee to keep them awake. As I had given up coffee, I just had to get through it without caffeine.

The surgery residents were so sleep-deprived they looked like death - dark circles under their eyes, and they were angry and frustrated all the time. I remember trying to get a surgery consult for one of the patients I had seen. The resident very curtly told me it was a waste of her time, but came down anyway. I had heard that she was notorious for being rude and was maybe the most unpleasant surgery resident in the whole program. She was terse and abrupt to everyone, which made me feel better to know it wasn't personal. But, the strange thing about her, though, was when she entered the surgical residency, she was rumored to have been very pleasant, "a normal gal." Since surgical residents are overworked more than the residents in any other specialty, it was no surprise that the experience had changed her.

What I saw most with interns and residents was their resignation. They were handling too many patients and couldn't keep track of them. Some were handling more than twenty at a time. Since the residents made all of the day to day decisions regarding their patient's care, having twenty at a time was quite excessive. One patient in an ICU could eat up hours of time, tracking all of the fluid outputs and the ventilator numbers. One AIDS patient could take hours to go through all of the medications to figure out what was happening with him since there are so many things that can go wrong with an AIDS patient.

The residents eventually came to a point that I began to call "the sighing stage" because I would always see them sigh. It was always about a patient who was on multiple medications, and it seemed no matter what the resident tried in terms of treatments or drugs, the patient's condition would not improve. They seemed to take on full responsibility for what happened to their patients, and a lack of improvement felt like a personal failure, which was when they would sigh. Yet at the same time, maybe even in the same breath, they would say something like how they were learning so much in this residency program and how lucky they were to have matched to this program as opposed to the other ones which were not as good. They sighed because they cared and because they wanted to help but knew they could not. It was learning about the limitations of medicine that was so depressing. We all thought we would be saving the world when we entered medical school. The residents finally figured out that what they mostly did was manage drugs and watch their patients worsen and die. It was a hard realization to make.

At some point, residents would finally hit a stage where this caring and empathizing with so many patients, too much stress and not enough sleep would completely overwhelm them, and they would shut down in complete self-defense of their psyches. To protect themselves from too much emotional pain of the frustration they felt at not being able to help, they had to stop caring. At that point, they became like the surgical resident - so closed off that nothing else could come in and hurt them.

The absolute worst thing about working in the emergency room was the lack of supervision. There was maybe one attending physician and possibly twenty students and residents seeing patients. The care of every patient would have to be approved by the attending. This involved finding the attending physician, and "presenting" the case to him or her. The attending would make changes to the treatment as necessary and sign off. All orders for tests, admissions, etc. had to be approved by the attending.

So, once I would see a patient, I would have to find the attending physician afterwards, and get the treatment approved before anything could be done. This used to turn into a fiasco because no one would ever know where the attending was. Everyone was always looking for the attending, and when the attending finally emerged from a patient room, he would be mobbed by the sheer number of students and residents needing supervision. Sometimes it became downright competitive; we would literally fight for the attending's attention. As it would take so long to get an attending, the emergency room would then back up, and especially on the weekend nights, there would be patients in the hallways, sometimes left there for hours because no one could get to them. I couldn't move on to the next patient until I had found the attending for the first case and handled that. I was spending too much time on my patients again!

Usually, after an hour, the nurses would find me and ask me what was taking so long. The patients and their families would complain, and wanted me to get them taken care of immediately. They would use a very forceful and demanding tone. Then, the residents would complain that we were spending too much time on the patients, and that we needed to be more efficient. I could be efficient all day long if I wanted, but I couldn't get the attending to sign off on my cases any sooner - this was the factor that slowed everything down. One day, I made a comment back to the residents - I said, "Just move 'em in, and move 'em out!" He actually took offense to my comment even though this is exactly what he was telling us to do.

It was too much to ask. I remember going home so many days, complaining to Marco, that no matter which way I turned, someone was yelling at me - the doctors, the nurses, the patients, and the families. I was in a catch-22 situation again. They were all demanding things that were impossible. No wonder my fellow students all wanted to leave early. It was mayhem.

There was a particular man who came in with a painful lymph node disease that caused chronic swelling and infection of his lymph nodes, especially in his armpits and in his groin area. The odor of this infection was very strong, and his negative attitude was even stronger. As I tried to find the ever elusive attending, I could hear him yelling at the nurses to yell at me to find out what was taking so long with the pain medication. He screamed about how we could be so incompetent, and what could be so difficult about giving him his pain medication.

A surgery consult was called in, and the infamous surgical resident yelled at me that this, of course, was a waste of her time. It was a good excuse – if it was a worthless case, she wouldn't have to take it, and she was so overworked, how could she possibly take another case? Then it was discovered that this man had actually missed his appointment to his family doctor, so he had come into the emergency room instead. Then, the surgical resident grew even more indignant. Everyone was yelling and screaming about how this man was abusing the system. It is medicine, the system, that "saves" patients, and in the process weakens them so that they become dependent on doctors' care, and then they start demanding that they be taken care of. Like little children, they demand this or that test, spewing out orders at the staff, "Fix me now!"

If you had a disease and you were told there was nothing you could do for it except take these pills, and the pills helped the symptoms some, but the problem never went away, you would become dependent on those pills to make your life bearable. You've been told there's nothing you can do, so why try anything to help yourself? Why not just sit there and be hopeless about it? Why not blame everyone else around you for this problem? After all, no one seems to know the reason you have this disease, which leaves you to think that you're just some sort of unlucky victim who randomly caught this disease. How unfair - why *not* be angry at everyone else because they seem normal and you're suffering! This is how disease affects so many people.

When I came home, I felt glad that Marco never yelled at me. He was the only one who didn't. He just kept agreeing with me and supporting me.

There were so many cases and so little supervision that some patients would fall through the cracks. There was a young lady who came into the ER with a vulvar infection. Over the hours it took to find an attending physician, I grew concerned, as it seemed as if it were spreading throughout her lymphatic system, and her pain was growing. I searched all over the entire floor multiple times, asking everyone I knew where the attending was, and the attending could not be found. I finally found a resident and begged him to see her. He was so busy himself, that I literally had to beg. After seeing her, he determined that she had a variety of flesh-eating bacteria that was rapidly spreading, and had she not gone into emergency surgery, she would probably have died.

There was a study conducted at Pennsylvania State University of nonemergency medicine residents. Cases handled by residents and then handed over to the attending for approval resulted in many major changes in care. Out of 1,000 study cases, there were 153 major changes and 353 minor changes in patient care. 17 changes were considered life or limb-threatening. "It is clear that a number of potentially life- and limb-threatening errors were made by the residents and

262   STOP THE MEDICINE!

prevented by the attending supervision. Our results confirm the importance of attending supervision of all patients in the ED...The residents in the study apparently could not distinguish those cases that might need attending supervision or assistance from those cases that could be handled safely by themselves" (Attending Supervision of Nonemergency Medicine Residents in a University Hospital ED, American Journal of Emergency Medicine. 13(3):259-261, May, 1995).

Because X-rays are mutagenic, causing mutations in an unborn child, pregnant ladies are not supposed to receive X-rays. It is a routine question before shooting the X-ray to ask the women if they thought they could be pregnant. The attending threw a fit when he found out that no one had asked this lady if she could be pregnant, and her fetus had just been exposed to unnecessary radiation.

The stress level was so high that working twelve hours in a row seemed like an eternity. There have been several studies done that show that under such high stress of making life and death decisions, that a doctor begins to lose his abilities to make decisions after just four hours. No wonder many of my fellow students would sneak out early before their shift was finished. One of my fellow students, a few hours before her shift was over, told me that she would help me staple closed the scalp of a lady who was injured in an accident. I had no idea what I was doing, and no attending could be found. One of the residents told me, "It's not hard, just staple it shut." Then I went to do it, and my fellow student told me she would get the supplies while I finished up another patient. There I was waiting and waiting - and **waiting** for her to come back. I never saw her again that night. Eventually, when I asked, one of my friends told me she had snuck out of the hospital.

Most of the visits to the emergency room involved either alcohol or drugs. There were youths who came in for severe acute alcohol intoxication. There were people who came in in drug withdrawal. There were auto accidents mostly due to one or more of the drivers being intoxicated. There were injuries sustained due to people fighting each other while they were intoxicated. A positive toxicology finding was the most common laboratory finding in the ER. Blood alcohol levels were always above the legal limit for driving.

Then there were the people who had no family doctor, and they came in whenever they got a cold because they had nowhere else to go. Since this was the county hospital, we had to accept everyone. In fact, the county hospital frequently would accept patients who had been rejected by other hospitals because of lack of insurance. It wasn't supposed to happen, but it did.

Finally, there were the homeless and the alcoholics. There were the suicide attempts - I saw a man who laid down on railroad tracks while a train was coming, and his friend grabbed him at the last minute. He had no idea what he was doing, since he also was very drunk. In fact, he had been drunk every day for a very long time. Long-time alcoholics would develop several complications including problems with the blood clotting. Sometimes the alcoholics would bleed from their esophagus, causing them to vomit blood, or sometimes they would have nosebleeds so severe they would require packing by a doctor.

What was interesting was to note there was an over the counter pain reliever, which if overdosed on, would lead to liver failure in about a week, killing the patient. I thought, *and that drug is being sold over the counter?*

Pulmonary Medicine

Powder, anyone?

In my pulmonary rotation, I saw a young lady who had had cystic fibrosis for many years. She was in her early twenties, and her lungs were so severely diseased that the doctors had given her a lung transplant. As we checked on her every day, I noticed there were so many drugs she was taking that there was a big list just outside her room to help everyone keep track. Despite all the wonder drugs she was taking, she looked horrible. She was terribly emaciated and could not gain any weight. The doctors thought it was wonderful when the parents brought her a pizza to eat. They told her to keep eating fatty foods to help her gain weight. There was no amount of fatty foods that was going to help her gain weight in her pitiful condition.

I don't know how doctors think it can be so simplistic as just eating fatty foods. But a person with a severe disease **always** has difficult digesting and assimilating foods, and they simply don't absorb what they eat. The cheeseburgers and pizzas only serve to overload an already overstressed digestive and immune system, and contribute to more fat and cholesterol in the bloodstream. More fat and cholesterol in the bloodstream makes it more difficult for the blood to circulate, making it more difficult for the blood to carry oxygen. This was her greatest problem! Every cell in her body was getting less oxygen and more toxins from the fatty foods she was eating. It was no wonder her condition continued to worsen. I saw the absurdity of feeding her body highly indigestible food, products that she could neither digest nor utilize in order for her body to heal itself. She was emaciated because of this and because her lungs could not support an adult sized body with enough oxygen. All of the cheese and dairy products she was eating were making the problem worse - creating more mucous in the lungs, and more constriction of her breathing tubules.

Another man came in with lung cancer, and he had already received several courses of chemotherapy. I remember him because he looked like he had been smoking all his life. He had suffered severely from its effects. His lungs were filled with cancer, his skin was dry and leathery (it looked like sandpaper), and it was also red because his body was trying to compensate for the lack of oxygen by producing more blood. He labored for his breath. He was hospitalized this time because one of his lungs had collapsed. This happens when a tumor gets so large that it invades the air sacs and collapses them, and finally collapses the lung. In order to keep this from happening again, the doctors performed a procedure during which they poured talcum powder inside an opening in the chest to get to the lining of the lungs. The talc would produce such a strong irritation that the body would set up an inflammation that would result in massive scarring. This scarring would adhere to the lining of the chest so that the lungs would be stuck to the chest and therefore couldn't collapse again. I thought it ironic that they were giving him this treatment because talc is a known carcinogen - it causes cancer.

Speaking of powder and the irritation it causes, there was a man who came into the hospital for a worsening of his Chronic Obstructive Pulmonary Disease (COPD for short) His lungs were also severely diseased from smoking. No one knew why his condition had suddenly worsened, until I asked him my thorough medical student questions and discovered that he immediately fell ill after powdering his dog with flea powder. That was not a good idea for someone with a lung problem. The flea powder is toxic for fleas - why wouldn't it be toxic to someone who was breathing it straight into his lungs?

I concluded that powder is not something that should get into the lungs, either surgically, or by inhalation. In my second year of school, we studied a case where a young lady died of severe lung damage and infection after spending the summer at her grandmother's house. She had been sniffing a powdered abrasive cleanser because it had a pleasant smell. It was a very common brand that most people have used to clean their kitchens and bathrooms.

After all of the disease in this hospital that I saw due to smoking, I saw a man who put my own denial to shame. There he was, sitting up in the hospital bed, when the doctors came by to check on him. He was in the hospital because of a pneumonia with a fluid accumulation in his lungs that had been drained. The surgeons were checking the wound where they had just removed the draining tube. He had suffered severe consequences as a result of his smoking, yet he told us that he really didn't think that smoking was harmful because he had just come from downstairs just outside the entrance of the hospital where everyone had been smoking, and he said he saw an old lady, "...just puffing away on a cigarette and she didn't look like she had any health problems." First of all, why was she standing outside the hospital? Was she a patient? Secondly, maybe her lifestyle would have killed him ten years ago.

In the face of experiencing a severe consequence of his smoking, he could deny that smoking really wasn't harmful. But there were others. There were the ones who had given themselves cancer of the voicebox from smoking, and the doctors surgically removed the voicebox to give them a tracheotomy through which to breathe and talk. And those patients would smoke cigarettes right through that surgical opening in the front of their necks. Talk about an addictive substance - there was nothing worse.

Next, a man who complained of a chronic cough came into the pulmonary clinic where I was working. He had been diagnosed repeatedly with pneumonia by his family doctor and given numerous courses of antibiotics, and yet the pneumonia hadn't gone away. We were to figure out that day that the reason he was still coughing was not because he had pneumonia, but because he had lung cancer. Specifically, he had bronchoalveloar carcinoma. The CAT scans showed the characteristic "snowstorm pattern" of this particular type of lung cancer. It was all over his lungs - obviously terminal. The doctors knew it was, but no one wanted to make the diagnosis until he had a piece of actual lung tissue analyzed in the lab under a microscope. They called it "Getting a tissue diagnosis". Since the man's previous doctors had missed the diagnosis, the doctors in this clinic went through their usual blaming routine of whose fault they thought it was that some doctor didn't catch this cancer early enough. The man would most likely have died, even if they had diagnosed him earlier. He just would have had more chemotherapy in his body and gone more broke trying to pay for the treatment.

He was admitted to the hospital to get the diagnosis. They tried at first to get a sputum sample from him, but unfortunately, whenever doing this sort of test, it is very difficult to get the patient to cough up lung cells. The tests was repeated several times before a good sample was obtained. Meanwhile, this man was sitting in the hospital, and the only thing the doctors had mentioned to him was that it might possibly be cancer. He was waiting with agony that can only be understood by someone who has undergone this same situation.

Meanwhile, I got to know him. He was a simple man, very sweet, and he showed me pictures of his family. His wife was nuts - literally nuts. She believed that there were people in helicopters over her house dropping acid onto her lawn, causing her to have burning feet. I thought, only a sweet person like this could put up with that sort of thing for all those years. It's always the cancer patients who are the nicest people on the planet. They let others walk all over them. Good thing I wasn't walking all over him, because the other doctors were.

They took charge of every detail with much bravado. The doctors had to do this test and that test and this procedure, and tend to all the details why. However, the attending saw him only two times during that week - once in the clinic the first day, and the other to give him his final diagnosis when they finally obtained the right sputum sample. They already knew that it was cancer that first day in clinic - but just needed to confirm it with yet another lab test that they had to keep repeating multiple times because it wasn't accurate enough!

I overheard the doctors talking in the clinic one day that they had received the final test result back that showed the cancer. They were talking like this man was not even a human being. They were saying that they had to tell this man that he was going to die because he had this particular type of cancer. It had never occurred to them to let me know so that I could be with them when they told him, since I was the one who was checking on him twice a day. The attending sat back, put in his short opinion and left the room, so as not to experience the aftermath. They did offer him chemotherapy, but at least they were honest: they told him that it wouldn't cure his cancer.

The attendings gave him the grave diagnosis and left me completely out of it. They told him there was nothing that could be done, and that he was going to die. I knew he at least had a choice. I knew that if he chose to do the work to heal himself that he could. But they got to him first which devastated me. It was at the end of the rotation, so I moved onto the next rotation, and I never saw him again. I couldn't bring myself to see the havoc that they had wreaked on him. I was brave enough to face my own disease, but not brave enough to face his, too.

Oncology

Indifference, Gloves and Caustic Chemicals

The cost of cancer care continues to increase from $35 billion in 1990 (Sondik EJ. Cancer control objectives for the year 2000 *Oncology.* 1987;1:25-35) to an estimated $50 billion in 1996. (Brown, ML. The national economic burden of cancer. *J Natl Cancer Inst.* 1990;82:1811-1814).   One out of three people are now getting cancer at some time in their lives. We are *not,* I repeat, *not* winning the war on cancer, but we're spending more and more money every year on dead ends.

One of the problems is our society's tendency to glamorize cancer patients. They are portrayed as heroes, their suffering making them martyrs. I'm not saying that they're not brave. They would have to be brave to volunteer to allow themselves to die a slow agonizing death caused by all of the toxic chemicals forced into their bodies. The cancer pain alone is unimaginable. What I'm saying is that subconsciously we know that if we get cancer, then we will get to be the hero - just like the heroes in those glamorized stories in the newspapers and magazines. We get to be brave and to have all of the attention. We get to be waited on hand and foot because we have "cancer." There is no incentive to try any other treatment.

The cancer industry is a multi-billion dollar one. It wants to perpetuate itself. It will use any tactic, any statistic - any means necessary to make sure it stays in existence. And why not? Why would a business not want to make money? What better way to get larger and more powerful than to convince everyone that they need your treatment?

A "Cure." First of all, a cancer "cure" rate does not mean a cure of cancer. It means the 5-year survival rate. In other words, it just means how many people are alive at the end of five years. It does **not** mean the spontaneous remissions. It does **not** mean how many people are cured at the end of five years. At the end of five years, many of these survivors are barely alive, almost dead from their cancer, or going to chemo for the fifth cycle, only to have it fail again. Or they are the ones who are just on large doses of painkillers, the ones who've been told by their doctor that they're going to die soon, and they are sitting quietly waiting for their own death - but they're still alive right now so they get to be counted in the statistics. It makes it seem like all of these people have been "cured" of cancer. **They have not.** Statistics can be tricky. They call the statistics "Five Year Cure Rate" on purpose - (a deceptive statistical trick) so that people will be led to believe that the chemotherapy and radiation and surgery have cured others and will cure them, too. It does not "cure" them.

People may be able to poison this particular disease out of their bodies for the moment. Let's not forget that they're robbing Peter to pay Paul. Their bodies are being *poisoned*. It will most likely come back in a few years, or some other disease will set up shop in their bodies because they have let it get so toxic and the conditions are perfect for another disease to grow.

These things will become known to you. Watch your relatives with diseases worsen over the years despite the "best" medical treatments available. Watch your friends. Watch your children. Let's go back to the word cure again.

There are plenty of statistics that show that people die *sooner* if they follow the doctor's advice and have all the cancer treatments than if they just do nothing. Doing nothing involves not bankrupting themselves with the expensive treatments, treatments that are so many times not covered by the insurance. It means living longer. It means not being subjected to medical mistakes and horrible complications. It means not teetering on the very edge of their sanity every time the doctor gives them the latest detail about the minutest aspect of their health. It means not suffering from dangerous drug toxicity and interactions. Finally, it means a more natural death.

One day during my oncology rotation, I noticed that the boxes of gloves hanging on the walls of the oncology ward were different than the regular latex gloves that hung on every other wall in the hospital. These were thick brown gloves. I wanted to know why, so I asked a nurse what the gloves were for. She replied, "For the chemotherapy." I began to understand why as I walked into the nurses' lounge, and there was a very prominent poster on the wall describing warnings for chemotherapy. It was very important to get the chemotherapy in the vein and not accidentally into the tissue. If it got into the tissue, it would literally destroy it, and the arm or leg that received the injection would turn black and die. There were other complications, too such as abnormal blood clotting in the vein and damage to the wall of the vein being injected. Not surprising, considering the fact that something toxic and poisonous was just injected into it. It is extremely important to inject the chemotherapy correctly.

I realized that the gloves were to protect the nurses from the extremely caustic chemotherapy. It could burn right through their hands if they didn't wear those special gloves on. One of the chemotherapy drugs we learned about in 2nd year pharmacology was one developed during World War I -- derived from mustard and used as a toxic nerve gas. It was used as chemical warfare then. Now, for some reason, chemical warfare is considered therapeutic. We're still thinking that putting a poison in our body is going to heal it.

After the chemotherapy had destroyed all or most of the patient's blood, the doctors showed concern when the blood didn't grow back. They had poisoned the patient so severely that their bone marrow couldn't make blood anymore. Then, they would do a bone marrow biopsy to see why the blood wasn't being produced. Many patients found this procedure to be excruciatingly painful. We would try to numb the area with anesthesia first, and then go all the way down into the innermost portion of the hipbone with a large, hollow needle in order to take a sample from the bone marrow. The bone marrow is in the center of the bone - nothing will numb that area. I saw this procedure repeated many times, especially for those with leukemia or lymphoma to evaluate the progress they thought they were making with the drugs, and also at any time there was a change in drug treatment. I talked to lymphoma patients who said they would rather die than to undergo more diagnosis and treatment.

After the chemotherapy had destroyed all the blood, the doctors used drugs called stem cell stimulators because they stimulated the precursors of blood cells to develop into mature ones. A resident commented on the exorbitant expense of the medication. For that price, you would think it worked well, but I was told it did not. I'm not surprised - they were trying to chemically force blood cells which had been severely poisoned to act normally. It would be like whipping a dead horse. Blood cells need nutrients to grow, but they're not getting nutrients - only toxic poison. It usually got the patients nowhere, or it made only a slight change in their blood counts.

One morning I walked into the hospital, and as I was coming up the stairs, I heard a blood curdling scream coming from a patient's room. This was such a hellish screaming that I wanted to turn back around and go back down the stairs and leave the hospital for the day. The scream had come from a nurse who had been diagnosed with breast cancer, taken all of the chemo and radiation, all of which had failed miserably. The doctors had left her with pain medication to control the pain of the cancer spreading everywhere in her body. The only problem was that the pain medications were all horribly constipating, and this woman had such a severe problem from this side effect that her bowel was in danger of bursting - it was called a bowel obstruction. She had not had a bowel movement in over a month.

I felt sad for her, as she had given her life to the belief that her medicine would save her, and now she was not only **not** being saved, but she was suffering unbearable pain. As they tried to control her pain with more pain medications, it became a vicious cycle. She would only get more constipated. She was not the only one on the oncology ward who screamed that way. I walked in every morning not wanting to be there. I didn't want to hear the blood-curdling screams. I realized that others had known the physical pain that I had. To see their pain, I had to face my own. I didn't want to face my own at that time. I just wanted it to go away.

But the patients wouldn't go away - especially not the most pitiful ones. One of my patients had full-blown AIDS. He was on at least 25 different medications. It was no wonder he was dying. I believed he was dying from all of the chemicals we were putting in his body every day. His legs were covered with Kaposi's sarcomas - I couldn't even see his legs. All I saw were tumors in the shape of two legs. He wanted the chemotherapy again. This time, the doctors refused.

The first time he had the chemotherapy, it had shrunk the tumors some - just enough to get his hopes up, and then the tumors grew even larger and faster. Now he was demanding chemotherapy. Not only did they say it wouldn't be effective, but the doctors also didn't want to spend hospital money - they felt it would be a waste since he wasn't insured. But the chemotherapy wouldn't have helped him anyway. The doctors tried to manage his medications, since he was in an extreme amount of pain.

No one could ever get his multiple medications straight. I spent hours trying to figure them out. I'm sure there were many that were interacting with the others, and he was suffering from many side effects of them all. If one were simply to look in the Physician's Desk Reference, one would see that that many medications are given solely for the relief of side effects caused by the other medications the patient is taking.

When I moved to Los Angeles, I learned about a

274   STOP THE MEDICINE!

group of AIDS survivors. They weren't taking any of the medications - they were healing their AIDS naturally. Many of them healed themselves so well that when they went back to be re-tested, they were HIV negative. I know of many others who had been in the last stages of dying with AIDS, and had been **completely** healed of AIDS.

Just when I thought I had seen the worst, I was assigned another patient who had been diagnosed with cancer of the gallbladder. He was an Asian man who was only 40, and he had a wife and young children at home. Every day, when we rounded on him, he was crying. He kept sobbing, "I'm not ready to die; I'm not ready to die." I didn't want him to die either. Who was going to look after his family after he left? He was so weak and diseased that I really couldn't call what he was doing crying - it was more like a faint whimpering. The attending didn't know what to do for the crying. She didn't talk to him much. None of us had much time, and I was totally overloaded with the AIDS patient - a full-time job.

She sent for a psychiatrist who recommended a stimulant because "the studies show it works." It was normally a drug given to children with attention deficit disorder. She prescribed and added on yet another drug to his regimen and not surprisingly, it didn't do much. Oh, he perked up a little bit, like he would have if we had given him five cups of coffee. But, she thought he was well enough to go home and die, so he was then discharged from the hospital.

As the gallbladder is a storage place for the yellowish bile that is produced by the liver, when there is a blockage in the gallbladder such as caused by a tumor, the bile backs up into the blood. The bile turns the skin bright yellow. To say he was jaundiced would be an understatement. I think at night, he must have glowed like a full moon. The blood test for the bile was called bilirubin and his bilirubin count was sky-high. Because it is dangerous to have the bile so backed up, the doctors had surgically placed a tube in his gallbladder that drained the bile to the outside of his body, through the tubing and into a bag that was taped to his abdomen. We sent him home to die like that. I often wondered how a person dealt with having these tubes in them, draining out foul, infected, cancerous secretions. Somehow, they handled it.

There was one man who did not handle it very well. He had been diagnosed with kidney cancer. During his stay, he berated anyone who entered the room. One day, the cancer ate away so much the bone in his arm that it broke. They kept sending him for more radiation treatment to decrease the size of the tumor. They lost. The attending physician wanted to put him on the stimulant for depression, too. It was starting to be the trend.

Another trend was to give a certain medication to increase appetite. It is well known that cancer patients and other patients with serious diseases lose their appetites and begin to waste away. However, whenever an animal is ill in nature, it naturally fasts. It does not eat. This is a survival mechanism that applies to all animals, as well as to human beings. Fasting heals them. It heals us. The animals also know, instinctually, to start nibbling on wild herbs. Now, you know.

Once again, medicine teaches us that we should ignore the signals that we get from our bodies. Forcing food into a system that is weak and cannot handle the digestion of it, only further weakens the body. When these people begin to juice fast - live solely on large amounts of juice - they frequently **gain** weight. Finally, they are able to digest what they put in their mouths, and they can handle the absorption of something so simple to digest. They can finally get nutrients into their bodies to begin healing.

I found it ludicrous that the medical doctors were telling the patients who were dying of cancer to eat cheeseburgers and pizza because they needed to gain weight. This is why they had cancer to begin with! Now the doctors were telling them to eat the exact things that originally gave them cancer. Their cancers only worsened! They still didn't gain any weight. They couldn't digest those foods; how were they supposed to absorb and use any food that they couldn't even digest? I was surprised that no medical doctor had ever put two and two together - they know fried, fatty foods are not healthy, but yet they were saying that they *were* healthy for people who were seriously ill.

Many times when I would talk to doctors, I would swear I was talking to zombies. They spouted off the latest research article, and what the latest medication was for a particular disease, yet they weren't able to use their God-given common sense and actually **think**. They had been brainwashed by the sleep deprivation, and nothing was going to "snap" them out of it. Sometimes I felt as if I was living a chapter right out of <u>Brave New World</u>.

We have to stop looking at so many hopelessly flawed research studies and start using our brains to figure things out. This is why I'm not going to start spouting off in excruciating detail about what this or that research study said about the effectiveness of chemotherapy. Read the following, and just think. It will make much more sense to you than going through the minutiae of the medical library, and looking up something written in technical language designed specifically so that a lay person cannot possibly hope to understand it. If you don't understand it, you become a victim, and much more likely to submit to these toxic treatments just because you figure it's so technical that only a doctor would be able to understand it. He's the expert, so he's using his own good judgment, right? I can almost guarantee your doctor does not understand the details.

Cancer chemotherapy, unfortunately, is not specific in its action. It not only kills cancer cells, but normal cells as well. Researchers recognize that cancer cells grow and divide faster than any other cell in the body. Their aim in chemotherapy is to kill these cancer cells by using cytotoxic materials (cyto = cell, so this means that it kills cells). Toxic materials will kill the fastest growing cells first. However, there are normal cells in the body which grow almost as quickly, and they, too, will be killed by the toxic materials.

The cells most susceptible to the effects of chemotherapy are the ones that divide and grow the most rapidly. These cells are the ones lining the mucous membrane and the digestive system, the hair follicles, and the reproductive cells of the testes and ovaries. Every cell in the body is affected by chemotherapy to a certain extent because these drugs are purposefully poisonous (to kill the cancer cells). If the chemotherapy succeeds in killing the cancer cells, what price did the rest of the cells in the body pay? Will you die later from the toxic effects of these poisons? It is not uncommon for these chemotherapy drugs, because of their toxicity, to **cause** leukemia or lymphoma a few years later on in your life. The second time is much more difficult. You may not survive because you have been poisoned so severely the first time and now you're going to have to survive a second round of poisoning.

In general, most cancer chemotherapy have these similar side effects (side effects would be a gross understatement):

1) Bone Marrow Depression - Bone marrow is found on the inside of the bones and its job is to make blood. This process is slowed down, if not stopped, by chemotherapy. Clinical manifestations include the following:

a. Anemia – a lowered red blood cell count leading to fatigue, dizziness, paleness, and shortness of breath when exerting oneself - even angina pains if severe enough. Because red blood cells carry oxygen to all of the cells in your body, you will be getting less oxygen to each cell. Since cancer cells thrive in an environment where there is little or no oxygen, you will be causing your cancer to **thrive and multiply more** by becoming anemic.

b. Leukopenia - a lowered white blood cell count leading to infections. White blood cells are a type of blood cell that makes up your immune system, and just so happen to be what your body uses to kill cancer cells. (Specifically, your T cells, and natural killer cells.) Chemotherapy just killed all types of your blood cells, including your white blood cells. So depressing your immune system by taking a drug such as this will make it more difficult if not impossible for your own body to kill the cancer cells in your body. This becomes very important because when you take the chemotherapy, it is so toxic that it will kill cancer cells, but it can't kill them *all*. As soon as the chemotherapy is over, nothing is killing the cancer cells anymore. This is normally the time when your white blood cells should be cleaning up the rest of the cancer cells left in your system. But they can't do this because they're dead. (The chemo killed them, and sometimes, they take a *long* time to grow back. By that time, YOU could be dead.) A long time ago, medical doctors used to use mercury to treat syphilis. Mercury is highly toxic to germs, and, when administered, it kills the organism that causes syphilis. But, it was also noted to kill the patient. They found out the hard way that mercury is also highly toxic to humans. Mercury is not something that belongs in your body, is chemo?

c. <u>Thrombocytopenia</u> - a lowered platelet count leading to bleeding. Platelets are what cause blood to clot. If you have less platelets, you will not be able to clot your blood properly, thus, you may bleed after minor trauma just like a hemophiliac does. Depending on how low the platelet count goes, you could bleed into your lungs, intestines, brain or peritoneum, all of which can be life-threatening. Again, you could die from the treatment.

2. **Digestive system disturbances**
   a. diarrhea, nausea and vomiting (in other words, you may likely retch like no other time in your life)

   b. ulceration - ulcers anywhere from your mouth to your anus. As you might expect, this can be quite painful. It causes heartburn and irritation of the entire digestive tract.

3.) Damage to hair follicles
> alopecia (baldness) Many times, the hair never grows back, even after the chemotherapy has been discon tinued.

4.) Damage to Reproductive Organs
> a. hypogonadism (your endocrine glands can no longer produce enough hormones like testosterone, estrogen and progesterone.)
>
> b. sterility (the inability to have children) You can probably guess that if your body doesn't make enough hormones, then it cannot make strong sperm or sup port a pregnancy, meaning that you will be sterile. Be sides, the chemotherapy just killed all of your sperm and your eggs.

5. **Carcinogenic** - causes cancer. Chemotherapy is so toxic that it damages DNA molecules. Damage to your DNA in particular area causes cancer. Since damage to your DNA occurs in random places, the more damage that occurs, the more likely it is that crucial areas will have been affected, leading to a cancer. Most commonly, the two following types of cancer follow chemotherapy. They usually occur 10-20 years after the course of chemotherapy has been given, but can occur sooner, and are not limited to these two types. Other types of cancer also occur.

> a. leukemia - cancer of the blood
> b. lymphoma - cancer of the lymph nodes (sometimes also called Hodgkin's disease or Non-Hodgkin's lymphoma)

> Eventually, the side effects of the chemotherapy will become so severe that treatment will have to be
stopped or the patient will die. For many of these drugs, the cancer cells will become resistant to the toxic effects through

many different mechanisms. This means that the chemo does not work anymore to shrink the tumor. This resistant effect is minimized by giving several drugs at once. This is why chemotherapy usually involves several drugs given simultaneously - called a "regimen." According to clinical results, resistance can still develop not only to a single drug, but also to multiple drugs. Now, you are allowing yourself to be poisoned by **many** types of toxic materials all at once.

Cytotoxic chemotherapy kills cancer cells by way of a certain mechanism called "first order kinetics". This means the drug does not kill a constant number of cells, but a constant **proportion** of cells. So, for example, a certain drug will kill 1/2 of all the cancer cells, then 1/2 of what is left, and then 1/2 of that, and so on. You can see that not every cancer cell necessarily is going to be killed. This is important because chemotherapy is not going to kill every cancer cell in your body. Your body will have to kill the cancer cells that are left over after the chemotherapy is finished. Now, how can you possibly fight even a few cancer cells when your immune system has been destroyed, you're anemic, you're not getting any healing oxygen to the cancer cells to kill them, you've gotten an infection because your immune system is depressed (yet another stress on your body), and you're bleeding because you have hardly any platelets left from the toxic effects of the chemotherapy? Doesn't make much sense, does it? This is usually why, when chemotherapy is stopped, the cancer grows again and gets out of control and grows even faster than before.

You may ride an emotional roller coaster because at first it will appear as if the chemo is working - the doctors will be able to measure a reduction in the size of your tumor(s). You may eventually find out that there is no way off of this roller coaster; it only goes down from here. There is now a vicious cycle, where doctors are trying to kill the cancer cells, and you're not able to fight the rest, so the doctors have to give the chemotherapy again, and then you can't fight the rest of the cancer cells, and then they give you the chemotherapy again, and by this time, the cancer has become resistant to the different drugs and regimens. This cycle usually involves you ending up in the hospital, taking even more toxic drugs in a ridiculous attempt by your doctors to heal your chemical poisoning by putting more toxic chemicals on top of it.

First come the antibiotics to kill the infections that you may likely get due to your immune system being destroyed. Then, when all the natural bacterial flora in your intestines is killed by the antibiotics and the chemotherapy, the Candida yeast will grow out of control in your body. They will keep wanting to draw your blood and culture it. The cultures will test positive for various yeasts and fungi. Then, they'll give the highly potent and toxic antifungal drugs, the worst of which is we used to nickname "_____oterrible," which, if you survive it, will likely put you into kidney failure. Then you'll be on dialysis until and if your kidneys recover. Then, the viruses will grow in your blood (by now, you have *no* immune system), and they'll add the antiviral medications - one of which is made from bat dung.

Pretty soon, the medication list will become so long that the nurses will make mistakes trying to remember all of the drugs and doses you're supposed to take. Then, you may likely have a horrible reaction because you took too much, or not enough of the right drug, or the doctor made a mistake and mixed drugs he shouldn't have mixed. Now you're covered with a horrible rash and you can't breathe because you're having a severe drug reaction. If you survive all of that, the doctors will want to repeat another bone marrow biopsy to determine why your red blood cells are not growing back after they killed them with the chemotherapy. That can be a very painful procedure.

After having gone through all of this, you'll probably feel depressed. But, don't expect to get any sympathy from your doctor. Expect to get an antidepressant or even the drug that they put children on who are hyperactive because "the studies show it works," and because your doctor is too embarrassed or ashamed to talk to you about it because all the treatments and drugs he's given you so far have been utterly useless. Although he'll never admit it, and it may or may not be a conscious thought, he'd rather you just shut up and stop complaining than to have to deal with his failure of not being able to "cure" your cancer.

The next thing that happens is that you may get placed on a morphine drip for the unbelievable cancer pain that you are having. You're sent home with powerful painkillers. You'd think that would be the end of it - that you'd just slip away painlessly? But, now, because of the pain medication, you're extremely nauseated and you're always vomiting. Not only that, but the medication has completely stopped your bowels and you can't have a bowel movement. This situation can go right into a medical emergency because now there is a risk of your bowel perforating because it is so full and can't empty itself. Now, you're in the hospital again, screaming in agony because your belly hurts so bad, and you're **still** vomiting from the pain medication.

The "en vogue" cancer treatment nowadays is the bone marrow transplant. This involves administering an even **greater** amount of chemotherapy that is so toxic, it's going to **completely** wipe out your bone marrow. So, this is why you need to have someone else's bone marrow transplanted into you (yours has all been poisoned out of existence). Only, it's not that simple. After the transplant, there will be a long period of time where you'll be in isolation in the hospital waiting to see if the new marrow "takes." Since it's not **your** bone marrow, now the doctors and you have to worry about whether your body's going to reject it, or in this case, whether the bone marrow is going to reject you. Because you have no immune system to attack it; it will attack you. Because you're in such a weakened state after all that poisoning, and not having any immune system left, that bone marrow could very well kill you! Or, it may decide not to grow. This period of time is tortuous, because in this state, the slightest germ that in someone else would only give them a cold, could give you a massive infection that could spread into your bloodstream and kill you.

Nephrology

Waiting For Godot

I quit my nephrology rotation early. By now, I knew I could do that. One of the first days, we were walking through intensive care, and stopped by the room where there was a lady screaming. As we neared the scene, we saw many doctors trying to hold her down and restrain her with leather straps. She was shrieking, "You can't keep me here! You can't treat me like an animal!" That was all I needed to hear and see. We later heard she had pneumonia, and she wasn't getting enough oxygen in her lungs, which made her delirious. They had to restrain her in order to give her oxygen. Legally, the doctors are allowed to use whatever means necessary in order to do what they think is best for you. The key word is **think**.

One of the most depressing places in the hospital was the dialysis unit. When I walked in, I thought I had walked into the land of the living dead, since all of the patients looked like zombies. Each dialysis session took 3-5 hours, and the typical frequency was 2-3 times per week, sometimes more often. These people spent a large portion of their lives in this unit. They were just sitting there, hooked up to the dialysis machines. They didn't even try to pass the time with reading. They just sat there with blank looks on their faces - waiting, waiting for it to be over. It reminded me of the book, <u>Waiting for Godot</u>, in which the characters spend the entire play waiting for their friend Godot who never shows up.

In order to get dialysed, certain immunizations were required. The reason for this, as one nephrologist told me, was because the filters in the machine were so expensive that they don't replace them after each patient. They try to "sterilize" the machines and the tubing, but people have still gotten hepatitis, the flu and pneumonia and other diseases which are spread through the blood from the dialysis equipment. The large number of immunizations made them sicker.

After about a week, I had enough, so I quit and moved on to Neurology.

Neurology

There's Nothing We Can Do

In Neurology clinic, I saw many neurologic diseases. One of them belonged to a lady with multiple sclerosis. Her symptoms were obviously those of multiple sclerosis, but the doctors wanted to make sure exactly what it was, so that they could target the specific drugs for her condition. However, in natural healing, if we can just get close to the diagnosis, we can heal it. There is no need to do complicated, painful, and potentially lethal diagnostic tests.

We told her we would do a spinal tap to withdraw the fluid surrounding her spinal cord to analyze it for inflammation and other diseases that affect the nervous system - infection, tumor, etc. The word "tap" makes it sounded harmless. We told the patients spinal tap on purpose because it sounds harmless. The medical term is lumbar puncture, but who would want to have a "puncture" done? No one would agree to it if we called it that. Puncture is more accurate, but maybe they should have called it spinal stabbing - perhaps spinal jamming would be a better word, since it involves jamming a large needle all the way through the skin and skillfully threading it through the space between the vertebrae into the space that surrounds the spinal cord and withdrawing the fluid that is there. If we called it a spinal jam or a spinal stab, then maybe people would get an idea of how invasive and painful it is.

The spinal cord is surrounded by the vertebrae. It is well-protected by these bones. This is why it is so difficult for the doctors to get into this space. Nature must have designed it that way for a reason, going to all of this trouble to protect the spinal cord from injury. Then, the doctors go in and mess with a very delicate system, and sometimes injure the spinal cord, causing paralysis.

The fluid that surrounds the spinal cord has many important functions. It maintains a certain pressure and is also continuous with the fluid that surrounds the brain. Withdrawing the fluid lowers the pressure in the entire nervous system. This is why people tell us that after having the procedure done, they had such a severe headache.

I also saw many stroke patients. They were all put on blood thinners or aspirin. Not a single patient received any counseling on why they got the stroke or how they could eat to prevent another one.

I saw the severest case of Parkinson's disease that I ever wanted to see. The disease had left the man without any speaking ability, so he just howled randomly. He was hospitalized because he had yet another urinary tract infection due to wearing a catheter, a device he was obligated to wear since he had no bladder control because of the Parkinson's disease.

His arms and legs were frozen halfway bent because no one had bothered to move and exercise him, and he couldn't move much on his own. He had rotted in his bed so badly at the nursing home that he had severe bedsores that were extremely infected. He had infection everywhere. The nurses tended to his bedsores, but it was hopeless despite the best antibiotics used. His body was far past the point of healing itself of any infection in the midst of receiving multiple medications. He was far past the point of the medications for the Parkinson's disease working anymore. The doctors didn't quite know what to do for him. They tried to decide the specifics of how much they should do for this man at this late stage. I wished he had seen a natural healer before he had ever started taking the horrible drugs for Parkinson's disease.

Intensive Care

When Private Becomes Public

Neurology was not the only place I saw hopeless cases. The Intensive Care rotation was the worst one I took in medical school because I never saw so much gut-wrenching pain, despair, and grief. Worst of all was the doctors' callousness that came from having to deal with such life-threatening situations on a daily basis. It became routine to see all of this suffering.

Each patient had his own room because the room was filled with all sorts of machinery that was "saving" the life of the patient. There was talk about many patients, one of whom had just received a liver transplant. The resident was upset because the man had liver failure due to being an alcoholic. He had another chance.

A few days later, he was dead.

So many people think that transplants are such miracles. I know it's a miracle if they even survive the surgery, much less the drug regimen they have to follow for the rest of their lives, a regimen that includes immune suppressing drugs that keep an individual almost constantly sick with infections.

Recently, I heard about another liver transplant story. A friend of mine, a medical doctor who happened to be open somewhat to alternative medicine, told me that his father had come down with Hepatitis A, and was so ill he believed he was forced to put his father in the hospital. Already, I sighed because if the father had come to me that sick, we could have done enemas, charcoal, algaes, echinacea, milk thistle, and probably some liver flushes. We could have nipped it in the bud. His father's condition continued to decline while I practically begged him to give his father some milk thistle, an herb with known liver protecting actions. I even acquired some scientific literature showing the use of the herbs in human studies proving their efficacy, and made copies for him. He was too afraid to do something that had not been established by his own profession to work.

His father deteriorated to the point where he was in need of a liver transplant. He began to have high fevers. Again, I begged for him to give his father a bottle of echinacea. You have to understand that my hands are tied when someone wants me to help a person in a hospital. I cannot get the staff to stop killing the patient with the so-called "necessary" medications. But, even with the toxic drugs, the echinacea very well might have worked, and it was **a definite** that it was not going to hurt him. Regretfully, he was too afraid to try it.

Another surgery was performed to evaluate the liver transplant, and the surgeons found that they had accidentally left in a stitch where they had sewn in the new liver. It had become infected, and this is why he had been having high fevers. The doctors had been trying to suppress maybe the one thing the patient had going for him, his own immune system that was creating a fever in order to destroy the microorganisms that were causing the infection. Again, I mentioned the echinacea. Again, he declined. The next thing I knew, the man was dead.

But, the doctor finally began to administer milk thistle to his father's wife who also had the same type of hepatitis, and she recovered. Ironically, her high liver enzyme levels fell gradually back to normal and she recovered.

Also, in the intensive care unit, there was the man I had seen in urology with the fistula, causing fecal matter to come out when he urinated. The surgeons had finally fit him into their schedule. He suffered a complication - surprise -

that landed him in intensive care with a severe infection of the abdomen called peritonitis. His wife looked on as he lay unconscious. She looked on in fearful anticipation, not knowing whether he would live or die, the furrowed lines on her face showing her fragile emotional state. All she could do was sit by him and hold his hand, not knowing if he even knew she was there. He was still there in intensive care when I left, although I heard that he eventually recovered enough to leave the hospital. He still had prostate cancer, and is most likely dead now.

There were many patients that we saw who had just had coronary bypass surgeries, and we were also taking care of heart patients who had been diagnosed with arrhythmias - abnormalities in the rhythm of the heartbeat. The patients wore special monitors that picked up the electrical signals given off by the heart, so we could monitor for any periods of irregular rhythms. Special receiving devices hung from the ceiling in this particular wing and relayed the signals to a room in which there was a large machine which printed out any abnormal rhythms as they were occurring. Someone was supposed to watch this monitor so he could immediately contact a doctor who could then help the patient.

While I talked with a resident about these monitors, he communicated to me that no one watched them. Shocked, I asked why not. He replied that the hospital couldn't just hire a person to sit and watch a monitor all day long. He admitted even the research studies had shown that the rate of survival is no higher on the telemmetry ward than on a regular hospital ward. I said then, if no one is watching for abnormal rhythms, why do we hook them up to the monitors and put them in this special telemmetry unit? It was much more expensive for the patient to stay in the telemmetry unit than on the general medicine ward. He said that they put the patients with heart arrhythmias on the telemmetry because hospital management tells them to. Period. End of discussion.

Around this time, I saw a patient on the telemmetry unit who wanted to leave the telemmetry unit. The doctors advised against it, since he would be out of range for the sensors to pick up the signals from the monitor taped to his chest. I thought how ironic that the doctors told him he couldn't leave, when it really didn't matter - no one was watching the monitor anyway! The doctors told him to stay to cover up the lie that there really was no benefit to having that monitor on his chest!

He finally went nuts; he was an anxious man - very type A. Staying on just one wing of the hospital made him feel claustrophobic, so he requested a leave from the hospital. He returned a few days later just fine. The doctors had grudgingly allowed him to go, but only after cautioning him that he would not have the benefit of having his heart monitored while he was away. He was finally discharged from the hospital on medication.

One patient in the Intensive Care Unit had been diagnosed with a type of leukemia. He had received all of the chemotherapy that could possibly be accepted into his body without killing him. The doctors didn't know why his belly suddenly started swelling up. They did all sorts of X-rays and blood tests, and they found some sort of bacteria and maybe even some fungus in his blood. Not surprising, since they had already killed his immune system with the chemotherapy.

His fever wouldn't come down, and the doctors were fretting over his swollen belly. The man was mostly unconscious and on his way out. Then, his blood pressure began to fall. This is one of the first things that happen when a person is dying. One of the residents said, "Let's try _____ medication." He asked me if I knew the saying about this particular drug, to which I replied no. He said, "We call it _____ - ed, leave 'em dead" (It rhymed) The residents joked as if they had just been talking about the latest football game. I thought it was a strange saying, so I inquired what the meaning of it was. He answered that the drug raises blood pressure for a short time, but then the dose must be raised continuously until eventually, the body develops a tolerance to it, and it doesn't work at all, and then the patient dies.

He said no one ever survives this medication. I didn't understand that. I asked, "Well, then, why do they use it if it doesn't work?" He said, "Everyone wants to hope." No one wants to see the patient die. I listened to the doctors tell the relatives that they were going to try this new drug to raise his blood pressure, and that there was a chance that he would survive.

In the next 36 hours, he was dead.

I was sitting in the nurses' station, a central common area around which were several beds of patients. I still remember the screams from the family members as they came in to visit him and were told that he was dead. As they wailed over his bed in their grief, I felt as if I didn't belong in their private moment. There was death among the hum of our most advanced life-saving machinery and drugs in all the I. V.'s, and yet, it was for naught. I felt as if I should leave. I almost did. I knew this was not the place for someone to die. This was not the place for relatives. This was not the place for patients. This was definitely no place for me.

I was under the supervision of a few residents, mainly one. This resident began to notice that I had a different diet than the regular vending machine fare and hospital cafeteria food that the rest of the staff ate. I guess when people paid attention, it was noticeable. I tried to answer in a vague manner, but he had me singled out. He began to make jokes at my expense about my funny eating habits and "natural" supplements. I resented the comments, and repeatedly told him he was crossing the line, but to no avail. I did not come to medical school to defend myself, but this is what I ended up doing. I felt like I was constantly defending my right to treat my body the way I wanted to, like I had to constantly defend my life.

On this particular rotation, it was optional for the medical students to stay in the hospital overnight on call in order to see acute situations as they occurred at night. I had grown quite protective of my body, and I no longer had the desire to abuse it anymore. This price was too high to pay, so I usually left around midnight. Pretty soon I started getting ribbed for that, too. "The dedicated students stay overnight on call," he would say, alluding to the fact that I had a "bad attitude." The dreaded bad attitude reference again. I just didn't want to fight anymore. I simply ignored him, and went home, only to return to the hospital early the next morning, still exhausted.

The tension became so thick, that I made myself sick. I had been on a steady detoxification, which took enough energy, but Claire had warned me, and I had experienced it several times already, that under severe stress, the body liquefies the poisons and they go into the blood stream, but they don't get removed. They "stick" and get reabsorbed, making a person feel even worse.

I began to feel the chest pains again, especially when walking up stairs. It soon became unbearable. One day, I began crying that I was having these chest pains. I couldn't take it anymore. The resident had my blood sugar taken, which was low, but since a nurse took hers right after me, and hers was even lower, he decided that I must be fine. He went ahead and hooked me up for an EKG, telling me that if it was normal, I was going back to work.

The EKG showed up normal, but I later found out that a person could be in the middle of a massive heart attack and the EKG could show up totally normal 30% of the time, so it was not a very accurate test. He told me to get back to work. I figured he had just lost his mind, and I telephoned Claire who said I was in bad shape and should come over right away.

I told the resident I was leaving for the day, and he was in disbelief. Doctors come in and work all the time when they are not feeling well. There is no excuse for not coming into the hospital. You come when you're sick; you come when you're well. If your EKG is normal, you come in when you're having massive chest pains. Well, of course, the lab test is more accurate than what the patient says, at least, that's what we had been taught for the past three years.

When I reached Claire's office, I was beside myself

with pain and tears. I couldn't believe how horribly the patients were being treated, and I couldn't believe how horribly I was being treated. I had finally had it. I wanted no more of this - I couldn't take it anymore. My words tumbled out, "I'm not doing this anymore, I'm not going on to a residency after graduation. I cannot do this to people anymore. I can't accept what it does to them! Can't we still work out something so I can still take over here after graduation?"

She looked me in the eye, "Does this mean you won't be getting a license then?" I said no, shaking my head, still crying.

She said that I could just forget our arrangement. She had hoped I could take over her practice, but she wanted me to get a license so I would look more credible.

Now there was no deal anymore. It felt as if my entire world just crashed down on me. That was the end. I had looked into several options, and all of them involved practicing medicine - preventative medicine, physical rehabilitation medicine, etc. The entire philosophy was so far away from where I was, I couldn't even consider any of it. There was nowhere for me to go after graduation.

There would be no residency. There would be no job. There would be, however, over $80,000 in debt. There was no job overseeing a natural healing clinic. There were no jobs out there for a doctor who did not want to practice medicine. I did not even want to give physical exams for other doctors that you could do if you didn't have a license. Why, so I could watch them slowly get sicker and die under the hands of another?

I went home that day and cried. I couldn't stop. I couldn't handle this amount of fear. The dread consumed me. I was alive because of natural healing, and I was practicing a form of medicine that is killing people. My conscience couldn't take it anymore. I couldn't hurt one more person. I just couldn't do it anymore.

What will I do? I'm near the end of medical school, and I have no way to make a living. God, I prayed, I have ob-

viously messed up somewhere. I just can't deal with this anymore. *Why don't you make this decision?* I decided to leave it to
prayer.

Between my broken sobs, the answer came to me so
softly - "Tell the story." Sniffling and hysterical, I promised
God I would tell the story. I didn't care what it took; I didn't
care what I had to do - I would go to the ends of the earth; I
would do anything. I had the precious gift of life, and I would
not let others die, not if I had anything to say about it.

Maybe not coincidentally, the next day, I called in to
say I quit the rotation. He exclaimed, "You can't quit a rotation!" In as calm a voice as I could muster, I paused, gathering my chaotic and terrifying thoughts. I said, "Watch me."
No, I would not stand for this anymore. Evidently, anyone
could quit a rotation - it wasn't a required one, and I picked up
a different rotation the next week. I subsequently picked up a
short cardiology rotation that was uneventful.

I could not continue to go to Claire's clinic. Everything stable in my life came to a screeching halt. There I was
facing the abyss. The seizures were coming probably about
once every week or two, and I was not even all the way healed
yet. The only other thing I knew to do was to try an herbal
program through the mail that I had been studying. I would
have to do it myself. I would have to take on the responsibility of being my own doctor. It is a common saying among
doctors that the doctor who has himself for a patient has a
fool for a patient. It was not recommended. It was considered poor judgment in the eyes of medicine. I didn't care any
longer what medicine had to say about illness and disease.

Everyone I talked to told me I was crazy not to continue after graduation with an internship. They said, "Just play
the game." The game was rigged. They were asking me to be
dishonest. Even my faculty advisor told me to put myself in
the Match process and then quit after I had been selected by a
program if I still didn't want to do it. I never wanted to do it.
No one understood.

I listened to the real doctor inside me - the one who

always knows the answers. Ironically, I had mentioned the same thing to the psychiatrist way back in my second year that I thought all of the answers were inside me. He disagreed. By now, all the answers inside me were coming out - they were there. There was a doctor inside who knew exactly what was wrong and exactly what to do. I would ask myself at first, thinking it was silly, but continued to ask myself right before I went to sleep what I needed to do to get healthier. The doctor inside told me, "Do not become a medical doctor; do not practice medicine; it is not for you." Sometimes we listen to this voice, and sometimes, out of ego and pride, we ignore it. But I already knew what the future would bring.

Meanwhile I took every last bit of my eight week vacation as I could spare and began the last chance herbal cleanse. I was doing things all day long like using castor oil packs, doing hydrotherapy routines, drinking down extremely strong herbal tinctures, exercising, and trying to get myself to stay positive about my body's ability to **completely** heal itself. I did this program for one month. At the end of one month, the seizures went away.

I made new lists to keep track of the long schedule. I didn't deviate. I didn't question. I acted and I did it. I was detoxifying very rapidly and I was on the floor again re-experiencing the toxins that had made me sick for so long. I had to make my own decisions about what doses of the herbs I would take based on how I was feeling. I had to just figure it out. It was all OK. The fear of doing it by myself with no supervision was worse than it actually was. I had that much control over my body, but I had never been taught to take that control - to take that responsibility. Sure, I messed up and took too many herbs. I never had anything bad happen, though, only more of a healing and one even faster than I had anticipated. I simply made adjustments in what I was doing, and slowed it down if I needed to.

To say I was fatigued would be an understatement. It was always during these trying times when I would get very clear with what I wanted out of life. I would get very focused about my desire to get well. Most of all, I got very close to God, as I was praying constantly for his help to get me through this. I was no longer blaming, but figuring out ways to love the minutest details about life, from clouds, to the grass, to my friends, even to my apartment. I was learning to love and forgive.

Although the seizures were gone, I was still depleted and exhausted, and figured it would be a good idea to do this program again. After the second month of cleansing, I realized that I was finally staying awake all day. I realized how long a day was when you weren't sleeping for hours in the middle of it. There was suddenly all of this time now.

I woke up in more ways than one. I realized the power of taking a risk. I knew I had to follow my integrity, and I had never dreamed there would be so much power in that.

No one was there to guide me or tell me what to do, except Marco who was there to say encouraging words and love me through it. He had no idea what the herbs did or what exactly I was doing, but he trusted me enough to know that I knew what I was doing. He told me, "You know I don't like to see you sick; do whatever you need to do to get well."

I didn't tell anyone else about the herbal program because I was not going to give anyone the chance to talk me out of it - not the doctors, not my friends, not even any other natural healers. I was living my life, making my own choices. It was my decision to make; I made it and stuck to it. Questions were responded to with, "Thanks for being concerned; I'm very pleased with what I'm doing, and I think it's all going great." When I said it, I really had to believe it. If I didn't believe it when I said it, then neither would they. I had to have complete faith in myself and what I was doing.

Then, all of the words of advice would come - "Don't you think you should go to the doctor? Don't you think you should get a CAT scan? You really should try this herb, this supplement, this IV vitamin therapy, this particular mineral, etc." Yes, even the "natural" advice would come. I tried not to get annoyed. I know everyone really just wanted to help in my time of trouble, but there were too opinions to process all of them. I had to focus my mind. I had to trust my doctor inside and do the one thing I knew was right.

Even my parents didn't know what was going on until I finally told them, **years later.** I had to be the only priority if I wanted to make it. Everyone would have to wait, as I was going to be so much healthier, more loving, understanding, and empathetic when I got to the end of the pain and the disease.

I learned that I needed to laugh and love more for me to get healthier, so I began to find humor in everything. Marco began to collect jokes at work, and he'd tell them to me when I got home. Even when they were stupid jokes, I'd laugh anyway because I was so happy to be alive. I would never take life for granted again. We would wake up holding each other, and I thought I can't get up without one more minute of just holding him. I loved him so much, I wished those few minutes would last an eternity. As I stroked his wavy hair, I thanked God I was such a fortunate woman to have him.

Whenever I was going through a painful healing crisis or an intense healing routine, I would breathe deeply, think about waterfalls and pink fluffy clouds. I cracked jokes. Doing such a strong detoxification was tiring; it took a lot of energy, but it was necessary, and I had suffered from my disease for long enough. I watched videos repeatedly to keep myself motivated. I listened to my favorite song by now - "Don't Give Up." Marco even helped me do an intense sweat routine. This was going far beyond the call of duty, but he was an extraordinary man, and he wanted me to get well, probably as much as I wanted it.

The sweat routine was considered highly controversial by the natural healers in the country, but it was supposed to be as strong a therapy as doing a juice fast for thirty days. A juice fast so long would be considered a very strong therapy by most natural healers. Since then, I have done a one-month and a six week juice fast. During a juice fast, everything that is consumed is in the form of juices, pure water and herbal teas.

I did liver flushes that were designed to flush out gall-stones, and toxic bile, fat and cholesterol from the liver. I blended together citrus juice, olive oil, garlic, and ginger, and took liver protecting, stimulating and cleansing herbs. I did flushes for my kidneys with lemon juice, lime juice, cayenne, maple syrup and kidney cleansing herbs. It was based on Stanley Burrough's book, Master Cleanser. I took an herbal formulation with echinacea in it. It made my mouth numb and tingle. It was a pretty intense tasting herb when the preparation was so strong. I took a chaparral-based, blood-purifying herbal tincture that tasted like turpentine. Not to worry. No matter what, I was going to be well, and I didn't care about taste. I can learn to love the turpentine taste. This was a minor detail.

I repeated over and over to myself that these herbs were God's special blessing to me and that they were healing me. I learned to like wheat grass juice and took other green grasses like barley grass, and alfalfa as well as different types of algae like Spirulina and Chlorella. I still take these foods every day, but not because I **need** to, but because I **want** to remain **this healthy.**

The castor oil packs were messy and I couldn't see the point at the time of doing them, but I was not questioning; I was just doing the program. They were helping break up congestion in my body's internal organs, a crucial part of the program. For many women who had used them on their breast area, the castor oil packs broke up the cysts and tumors in that area and healed them of their fibrocystic breast disease and other diseases. I decided to concentrate on my liver area, which is where most natural healers agree most toxins are concentrated in the body. I put it on the right side of my body in the front just over my ribcage.

The most interesting part was the colon cleansing. The herbs started the intestines moving and drew out all of the accumulated, hardened fecal material that was stuck on the walls of the intestines. I learned that it is normal and necessary to have one bowel movement for each major meal eaten during the day. To have less was to be constipated. While I was doing these formulae, I noticed exactly what the old natural healers were talking about when they said this material comes out. It looked like pieces of my intestines coming out. This hardened material was so stuck on, so hardened, that it took the shape of my intestines - it was like a mold of them. I passed this "toxic lining" with these formulae, even though I had been doing so many enemas and colonics for 1 ½ years. I thought my colon was clean! It was not. Enemas and colonics were evidently not getting in there and getting the old stuff out! Considering that water is a weak solvent, now I'm not surprised that it was not able to dissolve this hardened material and get it out.

I know there are many doctors who say they go in with their colonoscopes, and they don't see any material stuck in the colon. I beg to differ! Most people have an abnormal condition of hidden pouches in their intestines called diverticula. These weakenings in the colon wall are caused by many years of constipation - most Americans are constipated - and many of us don't realize it because the doctor sold us some ridiculous assertion that it is OK and normal to have a bowel movement, from once a day to once a week, as long as it's regular. The more people are constipated, the more they are sick, and the more they will require those medications that the industry sells.

A doctor **cannot** see these diverticuli with his colonoscope. A doctor can see these pouches only with a test called a barium enema - yuck - who wants that? We can assume that if you have a disease that you have toxic intestines - why bother with a test? The diverticuli are filled with old, toxic fecal material that is just continuing to get absorbed every day. The function of the colon is to absorb water. What makes us think it is **not** absorbing anything else into the bloodstream - like old, rotting fecal matter. *I learned that this colon toxicity is the major reason why people have disease!!!* Every good natural healer begins his patients with colon cleansing.

As I have guided people on many an herbal cleansing program, I can tell you that this is what I have seen clinically - people get well when they cleanse their colons - sometimes this is the only thing they need to get well! If they skip it, they stay sick. I know people who did this colon cleansing as part of their healing program for cancer - it was not colon cancer — and they passed colon cancer they didn't even know they had!

Maybe those doctors should take these herbs and see what happens, and then maybe they'll shut up. I would hope they would have a major healing from them, and then they'll think twice about saying to the public that they've got it all figured out how the body works (And yet for some reason, they can't seem to tell us why people get sick).

I was supposed to get into the shower and alternate water as hot as I could stand with water that was the most cold the knob would go. It was extremely cold. During these times, I would yell, breathe, pray, and promise myself that this was temporary, and somehow, I was going to learn how to love it all - even the cold water. I decided to try to make it fun, so I took my boom box into the bathroom and played loud music during the showers and I sang and yelled loudly.

How great it is to be alive! It was amazing how this stimulated my circulation. My circulation was so stimulated that I had this warm glow, and my body was red all over, even though I ended the shower on cold. I would almost jump out of the shower because it gave me so much energy. I didn't realize how weakening straight hot showers were until I tried it this way. "Wow!" I'll never take a long, hot shower again (without at least ending with cold water) - they deplete the body's energy stores and contribute to diseases.

After doing my first sweat routine, giving myself a fever which stimulated my immune system to clean up the foreign material which was still in my body keeping me sick, I noticed that I was feeling **dramatically** better. What an amazing healing routine! I had never experienced something so powerful! The sweat routine involved getting in a very hot bath with heat-producing herbs. You sit in the bath, and drink at least 6 cups of very hot herbal tea. It is a sweat routine, and boy do you sweat. When you can't stand it anymore, you have someone wrap you up in a white cotton sheet that has been sitting in ice water. (I was hot from the bath - the sheet felt really good.) Next you are taken to bed and covered with more sheets and cotton blankets and you "incubate" for at least 3 hours or preferably overnight. Well, I messed up this routine, too.

Sometimes I would do it, and I didn't get the fever I was supposed to get. The last time I did this routine, I got a fever of 104.6. When I read the thermometer, I thought there was a mistake, but I was really burning up. I just made sure to be drinking all of that ginger tea and I didn't dehydrate, and the next day, I felt really fantastic and the fever was gone. So sometimes, I didn't do it perfectly, but guess what? I still had a major healing from it. I learned that if I was waiting to do every routine perfectly, I'd be waiting a long time, and I might be dead by then.

I didn't think of myself as a particularly incredible or special person that I was able to do this routine. I figured if someone was very sick, they would do anything to get well. I looked at these programs kind of like a football player might look at his training at the beginning of the season - intense, but do-able. Any athlete would know exactly what I am talking about. You are constantly trying to push yourself and extend your limits. I was learning a whole new meaning to the word "limit."

I was learning that I really had no limits to what I could do with natural healing. The limits were those that I had in my mind - (Who did I think I was **not** going to the doctor? I'm going to hurt myself, I can't do this on my own, I don't possibly think I'm possibly going to beat this, am I? Maybe I should go and get checked by a doctor or at least a naturopath.) I learned to overcome those. I was my only confirmation. I was the one who checked my progress. I was my own doctor and I healed myself. Do you know how they always say that a doctor who has himself for a patient has a fool for a patient? So, maybe I'm a fool, but look at me now!

I could push myself really hard and even overdose on herbs, but I never hurt myself. I even took herbs that were considered controversial at the time - like chaparral and lobelia. They never hurt me, either. In fact, they are probably the most powerful healing herbs we have in this country. I attribute **much** of my healing to these very important herbs. Their bad reputation was manufactured by those in power who did not want to see people healing themselves. Too much money down the drain.

The first time I did the cleanse, I was trying to have it all timed out and written down and have everything perfect. By the end of the second month, I realized that there is nothing in life that is perfect - I simply must let go of this need for things to be perfect. I didn't worry about the dosages of the herbal tinctures, I didn't worry about how long I exercised, I didn't worry about how much water to put in with the tea, I didn't worry about if I was making the potassium broth right - I just improvised.

For, when in life do we have everything we need, all lined up and perfect, and planned out in precise detail? Doing this program has allowed me to be a lot more spontaneous in life. I improvise a lot now. Going back to a program with specific dosages and everything spelled out for me would make me feel like I was a baby. It would feel totally ludicrous to me. When I was first learning about herbs, I thought I needed it like that, but I really didn't.

I couldn't believe that in two months I got as much benefit as I did going to see Claire for one year. Keep in mind that Claire was an incredible natural healer and she helped people, every day, recover from cancer. But, the program I was now on was unbelievably strong! And I was calling all the shots! I was making the decisions, listening to signals from my own body, and I healed myself.

I went through an amazing transformation those few months. I learned to love myself. I promised to be kind to my body from then on, and I swore I would never mess it up with junk food or candy bars or beer or overly processed food again. I promised I would live my life according to my conscience and I would respect the miraculous gift of life that I had been given. I would take chances and I would live life fully without regrets. I began to be able to notice the details of life again - and I began to discover and appreciate what flowers smelled like, what the wind felt like on my face, how the warm air of the still night felt, the beauty of a simple song, the smiles of my friends, and the warm breath of my lover on the back of my neck as we slept. I began to hum, to feel my divinity, and to try to find beauty in everything. I wanted to see the higher way of life. It was all so very wonderful. I was no longer struggling through the day to hang onto consciousness.

As it happened, though, healing myself then began to complicate my life. I had never thought that healing oneself could have so many consequences, but it quickly became more complicated than I could possibly have imagined at the time.

Pathology

Is It Tissue or a Human Life?

During this rotation, I spent most of my time in the lab. The lab was filled with chemicals which I knew were contributing to everyone's illness, including those of the hospital staff. There is a joke about pathologists, since they work in a lab all day and rarely see patients, that they are social misfits. That was the stereotype. Actually, I found the pathologists to be very genuine people, maybe just a little too concerned with the details of everything. But doctors are trained to look at all of the minor details. Details don't heal anyone, but they made everyone look very intelligent.

Maybe if the diagnostic test is not too invasive or toxic that it harms the patient, and you have a good pathologist interpreting the test, you can actually figure out what's wrong with the person. Occasionally, a correct diagnosis was made without hurting the patient - physically or emotionally. It wreaked havoc on people to wait for the results of their lab tests. The funny thing about it is that lab tests are so inaccurate.

It was amazing what you could determine from looking at the cells and tissues. It was fascinating. The only problem was getting the tissue. Remember, I collapsed a man's lung getting the fluid out of his lung to send to histology so they could look at the cells in the fluid to see if there were any cancerous cells there. I was wrong to think that you could take a human body apart, analyze all its parts, and put it back together again, and it would be the sum of all its parts. We try so hard to analyze and figure out the human body that we've lost our perspective. We've forgotten to look at the body as a whole. Pathology attempts to take a part away from the body and analyze it as if it were totally not affected by any of the parts around it - a ludicrous idea.

Anyone who sees an anatomy book can see how all of the parts are touching and pressing up against each other. How do we in our right minds think that we can take it all apart, switch different parts out (transplants), take parts out (surgery), and replace parts with cadaver parts? How do we expect it to be a whole human being when we're finished? How do we look at human beings as if they were a piece of electronic equipment? Can we not be **humane** to **human** beings?

One of the reasons I picked pathology was because I only saw about four patients. I looked at blood under the microscope, and loved not having responsibility for putting chemicals in people's bodies. It was great to sit back and look at slides, studying them and learning the difference between a benign leukemoid reaction (a normal white blood response to an infection) and leukemia - a malignant cancer of the white blood cells. They were very similar and could easily be confused with each other. I learned how to spin blood and look at all the different parts of blood - the white blood cells, the red blood cells, the platelets, and the serum. I saw how the interpretation of a test depended frequently on the judgment of the lab technician, and there was room for error - many tests were not clear cut. It was not an exact science.

Not only were there chemicals in the air all over the lab, but when I walked into different labs, there were a whole different set of chemicals used to dye and stain, and make more visible the tissue samples, etc.

I walked into the histology lab where they do tests on tissue samples, commonly to see if the cells are cancerous, and I was taken aback by the very offensive chemical smell. I was simply horrified. The resident led me into a room where people seemed to be working normally, as if they were unaware of the extremely toxic environment in which they worked. I looked around to find the source of the smell, and I saw clear glass containers with labels on them that said, "Danger – carcinogenic," meaning it caused cancer. These chemicals were used to make the cells stick to the slide so that they could view them under the microscope. It smelled like a drycleaners, only worse. It smelled like someone had spilled kerosene all over the floor. These people were not wearing masks - they were just breathing in those cancer-causing fumes every day, day in and day out. I wanted to get out of the room as quickly as possible - I didn't want to get cancer.

The resident began to show me a different area where he got tissue samples from tissues that had already been tested. I saw as he brought entire organs out from the morgue in the basement, some from patients who had already died. I asked him, "How long does the hospital keep these organs?" He replied that they kept them for at least 4 years, as if it were something to be proud of. These diseased organs, filled with bacteria, pus, viruses, fungi, and disease were being kept in the hospital and no wonder people pick up so many infections when they stay in the hospital. There are germs galore in the basement soaking in what else but cancer-causing formaldehyde to preserve them as much as possible.

Formaldehyde goes into a gaseous form that goes into the air. Guess what I smelled as soon as I hit the morgue? I wanted to leave as soon as possible because again, I didn't want to get cancer. We used to joke in 1st year anatomy about the dead bodies sitting in the cancer-causing formaldehyde and how we were being exposed to it. It was no longer a joke. This was my body, and I loved it.

What pathologists are most known for is performing autopsies to determine the cause of death. I stood in on a four hour autopsy of a 4 year old boy. This child had been born with a congenitally deformed heart - he was born with his heart on the outside of his chest, likely caused by a serious toxicity problem that the parents had to create such a birth defect. The doctors did the best they could by creating a skin graft covering for the heart, and the child ran and played like a normal child until his death. I gazed adoringly at him lying there - his puffy baby cheeks, his mischievous, pouty mouth, his adorable curly golden hair that looked as if it had been kissed by the sun. His eyes were a gorgeous blue. He was so pale, he looked like a precious porcelain doll.

Normally, I would not have seen his face because it is standard procedure to cover the face for every autopsy, as well as for every surgery (except for surgery on the face.) But I requested to see his face because I wanted to recognize that this child was a human being.

He had had a life. He was real. He was not just some body to dissect and cut apart without thought. I suspect he had been the pride and joy of his parents. I touched his tiny fingernails, marveling at their size, and thinking that it must be the same wonder that parents feel when their first baby is born and they see those tiny fingernails for the first time. Except for his heart being on the outside, I could scarcely believe he was dead because he seemed so perfect - a wondrous creation of God. Maybe God put it there so that he could share it more openly with others.

As the doctors began the autopsy, they opened the contents of his intestines. They cut the heart away from the body and began to dissect it. All I remember hearing were the technical details about the heart. They were so excited because there was this particular defect and they could write it up in the medical journals and get published. They could take slides of it and show it in lectures.

They discussed showing the "case" to other experts in the field to see what they thought about it, too. They went on *ad nauseum* about the particular details of the various deformities of this heart. I finally just got bored to tears and, looking for something to occupy my attention, I started watching the doctors' faces as they were dissecting and discussing. What I could see was an intense discomfort at having to do this autopsy. There was an intense tension in the air that was relieved by all of the technical discussion. Then, I realized they were talking more to alleviate their own anxiety than they were about the child. It was disturbing to cut open a 4-year-old child. The way doctors deal with their feelings of discomfort is by intellectualizing them and talking about the minute details of the case - anything **but** their feelings. In this way they don't have to face their unpleasant emotions and thoughts.

The last of pathology involved spending time learning about blood transfusions. I evaluated problems patients had with blood transfusions from the most minor to the most life-threatening. If a person receives the wrong type blood (For example, if a person with Type A blood receives blood from a person with Type B blood), his immune system would destroy the blood, rendering it useless, and placing an enormous burden on the kidneys to carry away the waste of the killed blood cells. This could be life-threatening. For the minor incompatibilities, the reactions were commonly allergies or a mild fever for which usually antihistamines and acetaminophen were prescribed.

There were hundreds of components of blood to which people could react. This is because we are all so individually made that our immune systems have a very difficult time accepting into our bodies things which they do not recognize as themselves. There are good reasons for this. I believe many blood transfusions could be averted by stopping a hemorrhage immediately with cayenne. One should not underestimate the power of cayenne to stop bleeding until one has seen it work personally. If everyone carried cayenne preparations with them for emergencies, then when they came along, there would not be this long, drawn-out bleeding and the need for many blood transfusions. If people knew how to build up their blood counts with juice fasting and algaes and dark green vegetable juices, they would see miraculous results with their body making new blood cells at a very rapid rate - rapid enough to avoid most blood transfusions.

There was one man I was sent to see to determine the cause of his reaction to multiple blood transfusions. He had been in a construction accident where a truck ran over him and fractured his hip - a serious injury. The orthopedists immediately tried to do surgery to put the pieces back together. They knew nothing of cayenne or juice fasting, herbal poultices that regrew and repaired traumatized tissue, or any other therapies that would have brought these bones together again, including the herb, comfrey, also known as knit-bone because it is so well known for "knitting" bones back together.

After the accident, the man lost a lot of blood. Doctors don't know how to stop hemorrhaging except to find the blood vessels that are ruptured, go in surgically and tie them off. A lot of trouble, if you ask me. A good dose of cayenne is easier for everyone involved. Sure, it's hot, but no hotter than the sautering iron they used to sauter the blood vessel so it doesn't bleed anymore. After the surgery, the man started to have fevers. Because he had received multiple blood transfusions, there was a doubt as to where the fever was coming from - the surgery, the blood transfusions? The surgeons kept going in and revising the screws they had inserted and tinkering around in there. Every time you do a surgery, there is a bigger risk for infection and especially for fevers.

As I looked through the writing in his chart to see what had been happening with this man, I kept noticing the phrase, "Patient still febrile," meaning he still had a fever. They tried the usual antibiotics. They gave him two, then three, then they switched them around and tried all sorts of combinations of antibiotics, and still no reduction in the man's fever. Again, they were fighting this man's fever, where if they would have just supported his body with fluids and some immune enhancing herbs like echinacea and garlic, he might have easily gotten over this, no matter what the particular bacteria was that was causing the infection and the fever. But they decided to suppress his fever under the fearful, yet erroneous assumption that fevers are dangerous and should be stopped as soon as possible. Medicine doesn't recognize that the fever is one of the most important ways a human body heals itself. A fever activates the immune system; it speeds up the functioning of the white blood cells that clean up foreign debris and germs in the body.

Well, they weren't getting anywhere with the fever-reducing medication or the cooling blankets or the antibiotics, so they start looking for other reasons for this man to have a fever. Someone had decided that the reason for this man's fever was because he had an infected gallbladder. They decided to surgically remove it. Gallbladder gone. Mission accomplished. "Patient still febrile" read the chart.

The next thing I knew, the doctors thought he had a fever because he had appendicitis. Appendicitis? This man has been in a construction accident and had had multiple surgeries - you've got to be kidding! The signs for appendicitis in the chart looked weak, but then, they thought he had an infected gallbladder because of slight tenderness in the right upper part of his abdomen that might have been due to anything, including simple indigestion. They surgically removed the appendix. Appendix gone. Mission accomplished. "Patient still febrile."

I left the rotation in a few weeks and the patient still had a fever. But he had a fever because the surgeons were putting foreign parts in his body and inflicting massive trauma by cutting into the body so many times. It's been years since that incident. I don't know, maybe he's "still febrile." One thing's for sure, though. The longer he stayed in the hospital, the more infection he picked up and the more body parts he lost. We should make this a general saying in the hospital - the longer you stay, the more infections you could get and the more body parts you could lose. That way, the patients would all know what to expect.

After all the fiascoes of the third and fourth year, all of the crises, my own as well as those of the patients, it came down to deciding whether or not to train in a residency program.

I had traveled around the state looking at different residency programs. Everywhere I went, I saw the same thing. The interns (first year residents are called interns) all had noticeable dark circles under their eyes. They all told me that they thought they had picked the best residency program, and why this program was so wonderful - "The attendings really try to help you, everyone here is nice and patient with you, the nurses and staff are very efficient." But their eyes told me a different story.

It's said that people communicate with each other 90% through nonverbal communication. Everything except their words told me they were very stressed out, very tired, and very irritable, but trying not to show it. They wanted to know how they had gotten stuck here and now there was no way out - they had to come here every day, and go through the grind every day. And the hospital food, as usual, looked horrible, full of chemicals, and likely to make anyone ill who kept eating it. To see sick people who keep getting worse despite your best efforts is very depressing. In their sleep-deprived, brainwashed state, they believed the dream of medicine – that, one day, researchers would find a chemical cure for everything. They were going to wait for that day. I wasn't.

Once again, I went to the interviews. It brought up memories of the infamous first interview process to get into medical school. There were staff there to show the interviewees around the hospital, saying well-rehearsed statistics about the city and the hospital - the hospital has ____ number of beds, ____ number of these particular machines that save lives, it's owned by _____ prestigious company, and ____ number of patients stayed in the hospital last year, an increase of ___%. It began to get tedious.

When I listened closely to the interns' conversations about their attendings, I realized that they were desperate for more supervision, and that they felt like they were just winging it. The words dissolved into the air, seemingly empty and meaningless. No one talked about the patients except the interns.

I wondered how I would be able to live a lie for even one more year. I wondered how I could put the chemicals in and not let them know that they had choices - that there were alternative treatments that worked better than the medical treatments. I wondered how I could hurt so many people that way and still keep my sanity.

So, the time came to enter my top choices for residency programs in what is commonly called "The Match." The residency programs also enter their top choices for the students they wish to accept for their training. After several weeks, the lists are processed, and hopefully everyone gets the program or the students that they wanted. Wishful thinking, but it seemed to work fairly well. After the Match, though, there were a few students who usually didn't match, and the day after the match, there was something called, the "Scramble" where all of the students across the country "scrambled" to find the empty spots. There were a few reasons why students didn't match. The obvious ones were the ones who did not make good grades or get good evaluations. The others, although well-qualified, aimed too high for their qualifications - they chose a specialty that was too competitive for them, and they didn't list any less competitive choices.

I succumbed to the pressures of my faculty advisor and my peers, and entered the Match. I felt terrible about it. There was a long line in which I waited, one that led to the room with the computer. I waited there with all of the friends with whom I had shared so many experiences, the joyful moments, the tearful and hopeless ones, as well as the "I have no idea what to do, do you?" times. There were around 200 people in my graduating class, and most of them were there that day, making that line interminably long. In my mind I could hear the debate back and forth over and over, wanting a resolution, but not finding it. My hands shook and my heart trembled.

I approached the blank screen, acutely aware that I was creating a life out of the blankness. I could end up at any of these choices in different parts of the country. I sat at that computer and entered my choices for residency programs. Thirty seconds, and life would never be the same again. During my turn, I slowly, very slowly, I typed in my top choices, as if by typing them slowly enough, they would not show up on the screen and they wouldn't be real. Black words on white nothingness, so filled with stark reality. I did not want to make this decision. I walked away, heavy with the realization that I had sealed my fate - I had chosen.

I made that choice on Friday, but the final deadline wasn't until Tuesday. On Saturday, I was flat on my back in bed, sick and couldn't get up. Sunday was no better. During this time - my doctor inside screamed, "Stop this! You are not to do this! You are not to do them any harm." My prayers yielded, "They are my beloved children, do them no harm."

On Monday, I showed up in pathology an emotional wreck, and told the resident there, "I can't even begin to explain this, but I can't go through it, I cannot go into a residency." He had no idea what it was about, but tried to comfort me. I went to the restroom and ran hot water over my hands. That always helped me calm down. As the warmth went up my arms and into my body, I sighed, took a deep breath and made another decision. I had to be true to myself and my conscience.

I had asked for a sign - and it was screaming at me. I dragged myself to school before the deadline and signed a list that withdrew me from the Match. There were about seven other names on that list. I wrote my name along with other information including the reason I was withdrawing. The others were usually for military reasons. I wrote I'm taking a year off. It was a noncommittal answer, but I knew I would never go back. I began the task of trying to figure out what I was going to do with the rest of my life because it wasn't going to be traditional medicine.

Kampo Medicine

The Only One Enrolled

Kampo medicine was the only course on alternative medicine offered at our school. I was one of **three** who took it that year. I was the only one there for this block. Kampo medicine is the Japanese system of medicine, utilizing herbs and other modalities to heal. It had existed and had been used successfully for thousands of years. My professor came from Japan and his dream was to prove with research that these methods work. I hope he is still doing it. He had already obtained very encouraging results with rats, and also with people in China who were in a hospital and diagnosed with Alzheimer's disease. He was studying a particular combination of six herbs used in Japan which was specifically designed and balanced by an herbalist hundreds of years ago, and never changed. The herbs were causing the Alzheimer's disease to reverse. I almost went to China to do some training in this system of medicine, but decided against it.

The Decision

Dreams Do Come True

Two weeks after I withdrew from the Match, I woke up in a cold sweat from an unbelievable nightmare. I sat bolt upright in bed with Marco still asleep next to me and yelled, "Oh, Dear God!" In my dream, I had been sitting on a couch speaking to a man who was congratulating me because I got my first choice. I told him, "That's impossible! I withdrew from the Match! There's been some sort of mistake!" He was very annoyed and said, "Well, if you don't do this residency, we'll have to find someone else who didn't match, and the quality of the applicant won't be as good." I woke up in the middle of the night in a terrible fright and told Marco about it. I said, "Thank God, it was just a dream - it was just a dream, wasn't it, Marco?" It seemed so real to me, so much so that I was very disturbed with an eerie feeling that there was more to come.

It was getting close to the time when everyone found out the results of the Match. They would know where they were going to spend at least the next few years of their lives. It was a very exciting time. Traditionally a party was held every year during which the results were announced. This year, the party was to be held in a Mexican restaurant along the river. When asked if I was going to attend this function, I told everyone, "No." I didn't want to go and see my friends continue medicine. I didn't want to explain why I was "taking a year off." No more explanations.

316   STOP THE MEDICINE!

I had another dream about walking to a Mexican restaurant and sitting down at a place that was not mine -it was someone else's place.

The day after the Match party, I heard from one of my friends. She said, "Congratulations, I heard you matched at _____." I told her, "This is impossible. I have withdrawn from the Match. There is no way this could have happened. Indeed, for there to be a mistake in the Match is extremely rare. Finally, I had to go in and ask the dean's office what was going on.

Evidently, I had matched with my first choice. The dean's secretary had remembered every name on the withdrawal list except for mine. For some reason, she didn't have the list handy when the organization called to get the withdrawals, and she thought she had remembered them all.

I was in shock. But what was really shocking to me was that there was no effort on her part to remedy this situation, although it was her mistake. She told me I was going to have to go in person to the director of the residency program and tell him I couldn't do the residency.

So, I made an appointment and went directly up to the department to talk to the residency director. He wasn't there, but the assistant director was, a man whom I had never seen before, but one who bore a striking resemblance to the man in my dream. I waited at least half an hour in the waiting area on a couch, facing a long hallway in the medical school, terrified that I was going to get reprimanded or censured or something else horrible. What if he doesn't believe that a mistake was made? What if he won't let me out of it? My mind went all over the place. "Just shut up," I laughed inwardly, "Everything really will turn out exactly the way it was meant to."

When he finally called me into his office, I told him about the clerical error, and that I had withdrawn from the Match and was not prepared to do an internship. He responded almost exactly the way he had 6 weeks ago in my dream. He asked me if I was going to at least be in town next year, to which I merely responded that I would not be able to do the residency. He wasn't getting it. After I repeated this phrase several times, our meeting was over.

I walked the long walk out to my car, utterly amazed that my dream had just come true in almost every detail! I was shaking all over - was this really happening? I had heard that herbal cleansing and detoxification opens up your psychic abilities, but I just now understood it personally. Who would I tell; who would understand?

Throughout medical school, I had occasion to speak with an older student who had previously been a very success-ful engineer. I heard he had also made a lot of money in com-modities. He wasn't going to medical school for the money or for the prestige. He simply wanted to be a family doctor. He genuinely wanted to help people. His anxiety level was exces-sive, though, and the stress of medical school seemed to turn him into a basket case. Halfway though our training, I learned that he had acquired a heart rhythm abnormality.

The doctors really didn't know what to do about it at first except to tell him that they thought he was making it up. I guess he "appeared" mental to them. But when they did the tests, they eventually found the arrhythmia. He was on medi-cation and assured us that it was just a precaution. I don't think that anyone expected this man who was only in his 40's to die. But he did die from a heart attack, and it happened the day after he matched with a family practice residency.

The time around the Match is probably the most stressful time in medical school. You literally don't know what your life is going to be like, where you're going to live, if you're going to move the whole family, if you're going to stay with the girlfriend or boyfriend that you met in medical school, or if you'll both match in residencies that are geo-graphically close. The stress of it pushed him over the edge and killed him.

Everyone was sad for him, but I was not. I grieved, but I knew he was going somewhere better. He was miserable in medical school. He was constantly complaining about how he was being wronged by the students and the staff. He was constantly in a crisis, and it was medicine that he allowed to kill him - the system, and the medications.

There Are No Incurable Diseases

Somehow, I knew I was supposed to tell the story, and soon after I was asked to lecture on my experiences in medical school. I didn't want to do it. I had an enormous fear of speaking in public because when I was a teenager, I had to give a speech in front of hundreds of people and at the last minute, I forgot my notes and had to improvise. I considered it a disaster, and swore I would never speak publicly again. But, I was a brave woman now. I had healed myself by making drastic, very scary changes. I had turned down a residency, not knowing where I would go from there. I had taken about as many risks as it was possible to take, so what was one more? What did I have to lose?

At the seminar where I spoke, there was an herbalist teaching people how to heal diseases. This herbalist had trained under a master herbalist, a man who had taught thousands of people how to heal themselves with herbs. But, for all of his kindheartedness, and for all of the miracles that happened because of him, the master herbalist was repeatedly rewarded with handcuffs and jail sentences for "practicing medicine without a license."

I had watched as my conscience tore me apart. I cried for the tortured souls whom I was too afraid to help with unconventional means, for that might have meant expulsion from school. The medicine I had learned was not helping but was harming us all in a very horrible way. It was poisoning and mutilating our children. It was turning us into a new race of disease-ridden, prescription drug-addicted, chemically-laden mutants.

I had read many passages in diagnostic books at the beginning of school, but they had no real meaning for me. They were books I read for a grade. They were all just stories of misfortunes that fell randomly on unsuspecting souls. Yet, we as doctors were brainwashed by overwork, fear and sleep deprivation -- We became immune to those diseases, as we were the all-powerful ones - the deities. Our knowledge of the latest gene-splicing techniques, vaccines, or antibiotics would keep us safe. In the case of a terminal disease, we were the caring and merciful ones, blocking pain, yet firmly reminding those stricken that they must accept their imminent death.

But then, enormous emotions welled up inside me – the hatred, the fear, and the terror that I had experienced at the hands of the system represented by and contained within their pages. I couldn't let it go. Those pages spoke of doom, lost hope, and agonizing desolation. Yes, I knew the meaning of those words, for not only had I read those passages, I had **lived** them. Now, after having learned **and** experienced that there are no incurable diseases which pretty much made a mockery of my entire medical education, I felt as if I wanted to pound those medical books into the ground with my bare fists and bury them forever, so that they would never do harm again.

I had walked into medical school that first day, bright-eyed and eager to learn how to gain mastery over disease. I was complacent - I knew all the terminology. I thought that if I studied hard enough, I would know everything. But, in my impudent childishness, I had chosen to believe that we as mere mortals could fix the "mistakes" made by Mother Nature. But she, in her infinite power and wisdom, was not to be touched or improved upon, and she decided to teach me a lesson that has changed my life forever.

Sacrifice

Dare To Tell The Truth
To Save Lives

My parents were so proud of me at graduation from medical school. All of my friends were excitedly talking about this and that - anything - where they were going for dinner afterwards, which relatives were in town, all about the residency to which they had been accepted. I had nothing to say that day. Solemnly, I took my oath, and as I knew I was bound by my words, I sealed my fate that day. It was a serious oath. *Do no harm.* They taught us that on the first day. *Do no harm.* But I *was* harming, and I had to stop, and with God as my witness that day, I swore I would never hurt another living being with medicine or surgery ever again.

In medicine, there were no choices for the patients. They were not informed of any other alternatives besides the medical treatment. The alternatives had been suppressed and hundreds of natural healers thrown in jail to keep them quiet about the secret that we do not have to live with disease - that we have **that** much power to heal ourselves. And now, if we refuse vaccinations for our children, the school authorities harass us because they do not realize how the vaccines are made from toxic pus and blood from diseased animals and do harm.

Now, if we decide we don't want our child who is in liver failure to have a liver transplant, to have an emotionally devastating life for them and for ourselves, filled with doctors, infections, pain and ultimate rejection of the liver and death anyway after a few years, the government can take away that child and arrest us for "endangering the welfare of the child." Since when have we allowed the government to come in and take over every detail of our lives, including the most important one - the right to choose what we will have done to our own bodies and to those of our family members?

If medicine would have allowed choices, I would have been OK with it. I knew not everyone would choose this way of healing. I knew people would continue to drink themselves to an early grave, that they would smoke themselves into lung cancer and heart attacks. I knew some people would choose to eat hot dogs all day long, along with their doughnuts and beer, and not ever want to change that even if they would die if they didn't. But I believed that everyone deserved to have a choice, and that everyone should have the inalienable right to choose how they wished for their bodies to be treated. It's such an important right. We don't realize that much of it has been taken away.

I don't ever go to the doctor, so I am not in the system. I don't get harassed to follow some treatment I don't want to do. Whenever I have a problem with my health, I fix it with herbs and natural healing. I know what to do. So, I'm never faced anymore with these sort of desperate situations people tell me about with their doctor threatening them if they don't follow their medical advice. I talked to one lady who told me her doctor tried to black mail her because she refused treatment for her breast cancer. She followed an herbalist's programs and healed herself instead. She's alive and well today with no cancer. It's all about choices.

Doctors will fight and claw to the very end not to lose their scientific edge. They will try to discredit alternatives as unscientific and unproven. They will try to make us believe that each disease is different and should have a very specific therapy based on what the research says works. They will talk their fancy talk, and we will respect them because they talk in such an intellectual way that we do not understand.

Human nature is very predictable. We always fight the

changes, regardless of whether or not they will hurt us or help us. We are so fearful of change. It threatens everything that is established, and thus safe, in our minds.

The medical doctors will fight to the bitter end. When they have discovered that they are losing their patients to alternative medicine because it works better, they will try to take over alternative medicine. They will try to pass laws saying that only medical doctors can prescribe herbs and vitamins because they are the only ones qualified to do so. They will scare us into thinking that if we take the wrong dose of an herb, we will hurt ourselves, so we would be best to leave this sort of dangerous herbal medicine to the doctors. They will have us believe that we have no common sense to figure out how to use the plants that grow in our own backyards that have been used safely for thousands of years all over the world. They will try to turn the pharmaceutical companies into herbal formula-making companies with special patented processed and standardized herbs (chemically altered so that a patent may be obtained, and with a patent, lots of money can be made), and it will be about the money. It won't be about the healing.

This book may not incite change, but it was not meant for that. It is meant to be someone's hope. It is meant to change one person's life at a time by giving them the realization that they have the power to heal themselves. It is meant to help people make choices about their lifestyle now, in case they don't want to become seriously ill and debilitated later on in life. Maybe someone will make enough healthy choices to keep himself out of a nursing home, out of the drug nightmares, and especially out of the doctors' offices. There are so many diseases that even the medical doctors have admitted are due to an unhealthy lifestyle. Even the Surgeon General says that 30% of all cancers are caused by a faulty diet - one deficient in fresh fruits, vegetables and whole grains.

I tried to make ends meet after graduation by consulting with people on how to heal themselves with herbs and natural healing. I was terrified of getting arrested, as my teachers and so many medical doctors have. It was never a large clinic, as I worked out of my home. I had many successes. I also had failures, but I never, **not once**, hurt anyone with herbs. They were all only helped by them. But mainly, I was losing money because I wanted to help so badly that I was doing it anyway with no office, no money for advertising, and no marketing strategy. I could no longer afford to live on my own.

I wanted to move to California where alternative medicine was out in the open and more accepted. It was an extremely difficult decision. Marco wanted me to stay, but I was miserable there. No one understood natural healing, and no one except Marco understood me. I could not live my life anymore fighting and justifying my beliefs. I was so emotionally tired from having to be so strong all the time. I wanted to have my life be easier. What was I thinking? I already knew that if I didn't do a residency, there would be rough waters ahead.

I couldn't afford to move to California, but I had met a man at a natural healing seminar who lived there who told me that he wanted to start a herbal company asked if I wanted to help him? I was leery, and asked many questions. Evidently, Thomas was a big-time consultant for the multi-level industry, advising these companies on how to structure their pay plans, and how to become more profitable. I had even seen him lecture to one of the companies.

As we got to know each other, he offered to have me stay in his apartment, without rent, until we could get the company started up. He said, "Don't worry, the company will be great. We'll have your loan paid off before you know it." How much I wanted to believe this. I needed someone to trust, someone who believed in herbs, someone who believed my truth.

Marco and I went away for the weekend and had the best time of our lives. He went hiking up a special rock during the day, and then the sun was setting and I said, "Let's go." It was starting to get windy and the wind was whipping

324   STOP THE MEDICINE!

through my hair. The sun was setting orange on the huge boulder that had taken us half hour to get to the top of. I could see the shadows forming from the edges of the rocks, and he said to stop. There, in the most beautiful place in the world, he asked me to be his wife. I had already made the decision to leave to go to California and he knew it. I sobbed uncontrollably in his arms and told him how much I wanted to marry him but I could not until I could put my life back together.

Later, I broke it off. I loved him so much, I wanted to say yes with all my heart, but I knew I could not be happy in the middle of cattle country - I was the only vegetarian I knew. When I socialized with his friends, their main concerns were decorating their homes and what baby shower gifts to buy. They were always drinking, and since I no longer drank alcohol, I could no longer relate to them. I began to dread socializing with his friends because they were always asking me why I didn't drink, and why was I a vegetarian? Since I was new to this lifestyle, I had no idea how to handle it. It was so difficult. It pained me so much to be alive, and yet so isolated from other people.

He did not want to move to California because in so doing, he would be leaving his kids from his previous marriage who lived there. He really loved them, and could not stand to leave them. They were small children back then, 3 and 6, and he wanted to be there for them, to watch them grow up. He always had integrity.

I never wanted to leave him, but I had to go. I hoped maybe it would be temporary and that I could move back to him, but life did not happen that way. He had offered to have me move in with him and help me make my loan payments every month, but I loved him too much to do that. I figured I got myself into this situation; I had to take the responsibility of getting myself out.

I had to somehow "tell the story," and I knew it couldn't be there. There could only be one thing powerful enough to drag me away from the biggest love of my life - and that was my promise to God. I couldn't leave all those people out there in the world suffering so horribly the way I had before with my disease, and just do nothing about it. I had to do something. I could not walk away and pretend the whole experience never happened, that I was healed. I could not walk away from my destiny.

So, I traveled across the country with my car filled to the top with my things, and the rest of them in storage because I figured I would come back. I needed to be in California to study and learn everything there was to know about natural healing. Thomas promised that I could go back and get my things after the company got started. To this day, they are still in storage. Before the trip, I sold many of my possessions, including my furniture, for the money, and because Thomas said there was no room in his place for those things.

I had no idea he was going to lose his sanity in the next month. I don't even think he knew he was manic depressive, but he began to have wild mood swings. He threw tantrums, and the next thing I knew, he told me to get out because I had left two hairs on the bathroom floor. I only knew one person whom I had also met at the healing seminar and her name was Gloria. As he was screaming and throwing things at me, hard enough to seriously injure, I became paralyzed with fear. I had nowhere to go, and I was afraid for my life. Then, thankfully, he left and took the phone with him. To my misfortune, though, he took the battery out of the other one. Thankfully, I found another phone he had forgotten about and called Gloria.

When he came back, I apologized all over the place. I was trying to buy time - trying to figure out where to go. The next night he went crazy again, and told me to get out. Evidently he had had several relationships like this, and the woman always left and stayed in a hotel room, and then came back the next day and apologized and they made up. I learned that he had a previous girlfriend who had a child by him, but who refused to let him see the child. Now I know why. I suppose every woman has one story of the psychopath she went out with, and now I have mine.

He had sold me a dream, and I had stayed for the dream - that we would start the herbal company and educate people. As I found out, though, there were a lot of dirty little secrets in the natural industry. Every time I had suggested a company to supply the organic, raw herbs we needed, he blew them off, and told me we couldn't afford to start with those ingredients. What he was telling me was that the company couldn't afford to get people well because he wanted to chintz on the ingredients. He wanted to use synthetic vitamins, something to which I was strongly opposed, especially since I had seen just about everything accomplished **without** them. He figured the company should make what the people wanted - not what would heal them, and the public wanted vitamins.

We had met many people in the herbal and vitamin industry, and they had told us how commonly the major herbal companies do not get organic herbs because they are too expensive. One man had told us that when it says, "Vitamin C with Rosehips" on the label, there is often only a sprinkle of rosehips added - just enough so that they can list it on the label - and that much of the vitamin C came from the same chemical supply company - it was synthesized in a laboratory. Whenever I had asked questions about the quality of the products, I hit a dead end. Thomas wanted to continue, despite the obvious reason that the only reason I was involved with this company was to let people know they could be well.

I had read his irises and learned that his thyroid was toxic. Evidently, his father had had the same problem, had not taken his medication, and ended up on the street, insane, begging for money for years. I think he was very upset because during this time his father had called for advice because he was having angina pains and the doctors had told him his coronary arteries were 95% blocked and that they were going to have to do emergency surgery. He could have helped himself, if he had been willing to.

As Thomas had several months earlier sent his father

information about the herbs, as well as the herbs themselves, and his father had not touched them and was still not wanting to make any changes in his diet or lifestyle, I told him he'd better follow the doctor's advice because there was no way I could help him when he was out of state and not willing to do what I said.

Thomas' father died on the operating table, and Thomas never forgave me for it. I didn't get his father sick (it took at least twenty years of abusing his body for that to happen) and I wasn't the one who cut him open and killed him, but Thomas held it against me anyway.

Really, there was nothing left to stay for. He didn't believe in helping people, only in making money. He was such a polished speaker, though. He had me totally convinced that he really cared about people getting well. He had many others convinced as well. I later found out through the multi-level grapevine that he was regarded by his peers as a con man.

So I called up my new friend the next night when he flew into another rage, and she said come over. I had no idea what I was going to do. He was yelling at me that I was burdening my friend and that I should just go to a hotel. New to the city, I didn't even know where the closest one was. He said, "She'll just turn you against me." He was right. He already knew the routine - it had happened to him before.

She and her husband told me I had better get out now while I still could. But I had nowhere to go, I told them. "No worries", they assured me, "Stay here for a while because we're going out of town for a while. You'll figure it out by then." I spent the night there, called him the next day saying that we needed to talk. I tried to be as nice as I could to him because I was warned that he might try to do something to my things.

I went to see him the next day with the plan that Gloria and her husband would come with the van and help me move out in the evening.

So, I did what I always did when I had to do something I was terrified to do. I took a deep breath, held it and plunged full force ahead. I walked alone into the apartment where he was sitting with a poltergeist-like expression on his face. He had gone into a serious manic phase of his manic depression. His face gave the appearance of some sort of demonic possession.

It looked like he had stayed up the entire night cleaning and had not slept at all, but that did not decrease the intensity of his rage. Not needing sleep, hyperactivity and irritability, and even hostile and violent behavior, are all symptoms of mania. As a matter of fact, he had taken all of my things and packed them into paper grocery sacks, had stuck them in the corner and covered them all with a blanket so that they wouldn't look "messy." He had cleaned up all of the papers with which we were working to start the company, and he shouted that finally his place was clean. He told me I should be grateful to him because he had actually organized my things by sack when he packed them.

I was speechless. He said in a wild voice, "You wanted to talk?" His voice had turned sour, and I had no idea who this man was anymore. I just wanted my stuff back - it was all I had. I told him, "I don't think there's much to talk about; after all, you've packed my things up for me - you obviously want me to leave." He started yelling again that I said I was going to talk and now I wasn't. I kept thinking, "Has this man escaped from an institution or something because this is some of the most bizarre behavior I've ever seen."

I said, "Look, I'll be happy to move out, but my friends can't come to help me until this evening. He blurted out wildly, "I want you out of my life, right now; you're moving out right now! I'm moving your things to your car right now!" I said, "I can't do this in one trip - it took a lot of time to pack those things in my car the first time." He screamed, "Well, everything that's yours is leaving my apartment **right now!**"

Of course, I didn't trust him at all, and asked, in a very soothing and calm voice, so as not to upset him further, "You know, you've packed up my things in a hurry, and I need to make sure that you didn't miss anything, so won't you let me just take a last look around?" He shrieked, "No! You're leaving right now!"

So lastly, I requested that he let me call my friends to see if they could help me. "No!" he screamed. "I'm taking your stuff down right now!" As we walked, carrying my things to my car, he shouted, "You should be thanking me for helping you move these things! I'm doing this out of the goodness of my heart!"

On the way, I saw a security officer who asked me why I was crying. I asked him if he would stay with me so I could check the apartment to see if he had gotten all of my things in the sacks. Thomas started getting more upset that I had brought someone else into it. He said, "Nobody's going to believe this victim act that you're playing!" You're doing this to yourself!" The security guard asked me if I wanted him to call the police, and at first I said no, until Thomas's behavior kept getting more bizarre and hostile, and I was afraid for my life again.

Thomas said, "If you call the police, they'll never believe you! They'll tell you to get out because it's **my** apartment. I said, "Call the police" and the guard called the police, who then assisted me in retrieving the VCR and a whole closet full of clothes, along with many other things Thomas had conveniently forgotten to pack. The police tried to reason with him, and Thomas just kept repeating the same nonsense over and over again. The police couldn't make any sense out of him, either.

So, there I was in the parking lot, for hours waiting for my friends to pick me up because I had never gotten the chance to call them. The police offered to stay with me for the first few hours. Not everything would fit in the car, and so things were just piled up around it, and I was standing there amidst all of the things I possessed with my life in full view of everyone. If there was ever a moment to be embarrassed, that was it. The policeman told me never to go back to this abusive man. I said, "Don't worry."

Finally, Gloria and her husband Jonathan showed up and we packed everything that wouldn't fit in my car into their van. Their apartment was a one-bedroom, so there was no room for my things there. Half stayed in my car, and half went into storage. I prayed my car wouldn't get stolen.

Now I had to decide all over again what to do with my life. No money, no plan, wanting to help people, and needing to tell the story -- somehow. It seemed hopeless and ridiculous.

Gloria, Jonathan and I spent time together doing yoga and meditation, as they were yogis, as well as entertainers. They taught me all about raw and living foods. They juiced wheatgrass and ate lots of sprouts. They taught me how to breathe and stretch and meditate, and gave me lots of kava kava, and an herbal formula called "Herbal Proz" to help me with my dire emotional situation.

I was in shock for months, and could not shake myself out of it. But the herbs helped me through it. It would have been easier if Thomas hadn't been leaving me thirty minute long messages on my voicemail wanting to get back together, and sending me long letters and gifts. He did this for 8 months, ignoring my demands to leave me alone, until I finally threatened him with a restraining order and changed my number. I believe he was very familiar with that routine, so he backed off immediately. It would have been nice to know all of this history about this man before, but I made a rushed and impetuous decision, and I got to experience the consequences of that decision.

What I enjoyed most were the hikes that the three of us would go on in the Hollywood hills. After they left to go on their trip, they told me that I could probably hike alone there because it was pretty safe, and they rarely saw anyone there.

I left one day to go hiking in the hills. There was one trail leading to the top, and it took about half an hour of fast walking to get to the top. There was another trail that started at the top that went around the tops of the hills. We had hiked that trail once, and it had taken us about three hours.

I was going to get my head together and decide what to do in the midst of a city where I knew few people and had no resources. I found a rock at the top of the hill, and I sat down, closed my eyes and began to meditate. The sun was very warm that day, and there was a gentle breeze that lulled me into a very relaxed state.

All of a sudden, I heard a rustling noise, which didn't seem to concern me, but I opened my eyes nonetheless. I had seen no one on the way up. No problem, just another hiker. This hiker was naked and squatted down beside me to ask me if he could jerk off while he was watching me. As I screamed, he gripped both of my arms, as if by a vise, and I could not get free. He was young, muscular and strong, and from his haircut, looked as if he was in the military. I shouted silently in my head as visions of my dead body thrown over the side of the hill never to be found leaped in front of my eyes, "I'm not going to die, not after all I have been through! I have **not** told the story yet! I am **NOT** leaving!!! - do you hear me, God?! - I... mean...it!"

I had taken karate years ago, but couldn't seem to re-member anything in the moment of panic except how to scream. He kept saying over and over, "Don't worry, I won't hurtcha, I won't hurtcha." His eyes were lying - I didn't be-lieve him for one second. I kept pulling against his grip with all of my 100 pounds, and I was able to get right in his face where I screamed like bloody murder as loud as I could. I gasped for another full breath, and screamed again. I got an-other breath, and another one, and another one, and many more.

I could see his hazel eyes were filled with a stone cold detachment as if this were a normal everyday activity for him. We were eye to eye, and I was screaming my most ferocious screams as if to tell him, "I am going to fight you tooth and nail, mister, every minute you hold onto me, and I will not stop!" I would have fought to the bitter end. Thank God he was naked, and had nowhere to put a weapon. I had a mission, and I was not ready to leave this planet.

Miraculously, he let me go. He walked away saying he was sorry, and to please not tell anyone about this. "But," he added, "I was here first, and you were the one who disturbed me!" As he started walking towards me again, I screamed, "Get away from me right now!" and he turned to walk away, and again turned around, started walking toward me and addressed me, and I bellowed out again, "Get away from me!"

He began to walk back down the trail, which was the short, half hour way down. And I watched him go, noticing that there was not another soul around. I thought, I'll have to wait for him to get to the bottom before I can go down. But then, I thought *he could hide in the bushes and attack me again if I go down that way!* I could barely see him walking along the trail because of the brush in the way. I had no way of knowing if and when he got to the bottom.

I knew that I would have to take the long three-hour way which had a different end destination, and I would have to remember how to do it from only having hiked it once. I began to run. I knew when he noticed I wasn't there, he could turn around and follow me, so I was in a race against him, running and constantly checking my back. I ran up hills and rocks that I didn't think I normally could have done. Sweating and tired from the heat - it was noon - I kept going until I had gotten myself thoroughly lost. The trail was not marked well, and parts of it were overgrown. I pushed myself through some brush and found a construction site. It was not the end of the trail, but maybe someone was there. I checked every building until I found some men working. They called the police. Again, the police. I had never before Thomas had to call the police. The police and I tried to find the man that day, but couldn't. They told me the best they could do was to have me call 911 if I ever saw the man again. This was Los Angeles. Welcome, Dr. Foster.

Maybe I should have left Los Angeles then, but I was there for a reason, and I would not give up. I eventually found a job at a health food store where I urged people to clean up their diets, their colons, and take their greens instead of the vitamins and other expensive "magic bullets" that didn't work. After a while, I could afford to rent a place, and I moved out of Gloria and Jonathan's apartment and have missed them terribly ever since.

Slowly, I began to build myself another life. Marco and I tried to get together several times, and I wanted to be with him so badly, but I just couldn't make it in Los Angeles yet. I was scraping for every penny. I wasn't finished yet. Our short times together were so wonderful, but so gut-wrenching for both of us when he would leave.

He got to see me do my first speaking gig for a company representing herbal products. The pay was horrible, and the attitude was cheap, but it was a living, and somehow I was going to tell this story. They let me talk and gave me an audience.

I came to the realization that this story was to be a book, but I was not a writer. I had no one to commission me to write it. I had to pound it out myself in my spare time when I was not working, and I no more wanted to do it than I wanted to speak in public that first time. But it had to be done.

I learned so many things from living in Los Angeles. First, take a self-defense class. Second, never hike alone. Third, you get out of this life exactly what you're supposed to get out of it. Four, it doesn't really matter what you do, it's your attitude that matters while you're doing it. Fifth, we can't presume to think that because we have found a way to heal, that everyone will want to do it. And sixth, we can't expect everyone to be the same as us or make the same choices as we do in life.

Sometimes people travel down this natural healing path, and they never come back and they keep going farther away, all the while telling everyone else that they are wrong - you're wrong for not being a vegetarian, you're wrong for taking antibiotics, you're wrong for vaccinating your children. All of these things have consequences, but these actions are not for us to judge. We are here for each other, without exception.

Although medical school was the most difficult thing that happened to me, I am not sorry that I went. I'm not sorry I went to the doctors; there were many things I had to learn by going there and not getting help. I had a greater purpose. There is no way to know what life will bring us. We can't know the future. Besides, it would take all of the fun and adventure out of it. And life is always an adventure.

One adventure I had trouble accepting was when my car was totaled by a lady who ran a red light. Oh, you ask, how is the whiplash? I'll tell you. The first few days, I figured it was no problem and that I wouldn't fast. That was a bad idea. I couldn't move my back or neck for one week. The pain began to improve after a few days, but after a week, I decided to get serious. I went to San Diego to a chiropractor who does something called Neuro-Cranial Restructuring. I immediately began to juice fast. I took strong tinctures of kava kava and lobelia and wild yam, all known for their antispasmodic effects. After four days of his treatments, I could move my back and neck again - a miracle. I continued with large doses of algaes and cereal grasses to help my body build new tissue. He continued to put my bones back into their proper place, including a few ribs and a dislocated shoulder.

The chiropractor worked with a massage therapist who gave very deep massages. This man massaged the heck out of my back and all the muscles contributing to the whiplash. I yelled. I screamed. I cried. I prayed. The massage therapist taught me how to give myself a deep massage by rolling on tennis balls. OWWW! I did these deep massages on myself every day. I took a Rambo-like attitude and did not stop until all traces of the whiplash were gone. I did alternating hot and cold showers on my neck and back to increase circulation there. I took an herbal formula called Bone, Flesh and Cartilage to regenerate - you guessed it - my bone, flesh, and cartilage. I took lots of cayenne, again for stimulating the circulation. I rubbed an herbal healing oil all over my back right after the showers, and I found out how intense things like peppermint oil and cayenne can be afterwards. All of those things worked very well. It's all gone. My back is better than before I had the accident. I forgave the lady who ran the red light. I guess it's a good thing I had the accident. It gave me the opportunity to heal my back which had been so damaged from all of those years of having seizures. It took about one and a half months.

I heard other stories about how people had become disabled with arthritis after their whiplash. I heard about the chronic disc problems afterwards. I used to see those patients during my family practice rotation. Many had horrible whiplash pain that took months and sometimes years to get rid of. Not me. Mine was considered severe, and I also was having disc symptoms - nerve pains shooting down the backs of my legs, but it's gone now. To tell you the truth, I had no idea I could heal it. I believed in the theory. I knew it was a possibility. I just didn't know what I was capable of doing until I tried. Look at what happens when we try!

The Meaning of Disease

I thought that disease was the enemy. When the doctors said I had some mental disorder, I was so willing to accept I was defective and worthless. I thought I was my pain. I thought I was my disease. When I saw people healed of their diseases and I healed mine, I thought healing the disease was fixing the problem. And then when I'd hear stories of other people talking about their trauma because their relative was terminally ill, I thought they would never have that trauma if their relative had healed with natural healing. I thought that would fix it. But the truth is they would still have the trauma.

My disease was my excuse not to get close to people. But that story started a long time ago, long before I ever got sick. I told myself the story, "I'm all alone in this world; I have to make it on my own." I sentenced myself to live that out for the rest of my life, based on the decision I made about life when I was three years old. I made a decision based not on reality, but on the inner workings of the brain of a 3-year-old child.

When I was sick, it was the **experience** of being sick that was so traumatic, not the sickness itself. The pain was horrible, but I've realized that we are human beings having experiences. We have experiences of love, of joy, of pain, of disease, but we are not those experiences. We are not our diseases. We are not our pain. When I was so ill, people would ask if they could help me, and I would tell them , "No!" or "No, I can't see you because I don't want you to see me this way!" Really, my disease was just another excuse for me to be a victim, all alone, suffering with no one caring about me. I never gave anyone the real opportunity to help me. I always kept everyone at arm's length.

I kept asking my nutritionist, "When am I going to be healed?" because I thought all of my problems would be solved if I were only healed of my disease. I was asking the wrong question. I should have been asking, "When am I going to accept who I am right now exactly the way I am - sick or not sick?"

When I saw patients suffering, I still thought disease was the enemy. I saw them in pain, and I thought they were the pain and the disease just as I knew I was the pain and the disease. So I thought if I could fix their disease, all the pain would go away.

I moved all the way across the country. I left a man who loved me and wanted to marry me because I thought disease was the enemy. I went in search of the cures for incurable diseases, and I found them. But that was never the point. The point was my pain, my solitude that I had decided on as a young child and didn't know better than to keep recreating it over the years in different ways, including the experience of having a disease. I realize now I no longer have to fix people's diseases because disease is not the enemy. If they were not having the experience of having a disease, they would be having an equally painful experience except that would not involve a disease. It would be something else that would make them suffer emotionally in a similar way.

I had to ask myself why, although I was healed, did I still feel alone? I was healed, so disease was no longer my excuse for being alone. I worked all day, then I came home and I worked all night, and when someone asked me to do something, I told them, "I'm too busy - I can't do it." I didn't realize suffering was in the mind, not in the body. This is why I still felt so alone and my life was in such chaos even after I healed my disease. I had to finally find peace of mind and learn how to stop creating chaos. I had to come full circle before I finally found peace. It is not anything outside of ourselves - medicine or even herbs - that can heal our lives. It is that miraculous power within us that can heal anything. Now I have my healing **and** my peace.

There are saints and mystics who take on diseases, but they do not suffer because of them. The disease has no meaning to them. The pain has no meaning to them. The disease did not mean to them that they were being punished, that they were defective in some way, that their spouse was going to leave them, that they were going to lose their job, that they weren't going to be able to do certain activities anymore, that they would have to be dependent on others to help them. There are no meanings at all to disease except those that we superimpose upon it. This was the issue.

People always say, don't make waves. They might as well say, "It's not safe to be yourself." I've learned that it is more dangerous **not** to be who you are. It **is** safe to be exactly who you are -- fully. If I can do what I've done, then you can do **anything!!!**

As for me, I'm living my life fully without regrets. I speak my mind out of love for others, without worry for the consequences. If I need to make waves in order to make life easier, to ease suffering, to end pain, I will do it -- **without hesitation**. I will give my love until there is none left to give, but I will always have more to give. I'm alive. I can walk. I can talk. What's more - I can dance, and I can sing, and I can

338   STOP THE MEDICINE!

love. And I have **so** many thoughts now that they fill my head and spill over onto the pages. I have the ability to tell this story. I will always give thanks for these things. I have fulfilled my promise - I told the story, and I hope that after reading this book, your life will be as changed in as beautiful and as exciting a way as it has been for me. And what a beautiful, irreplaceable gift that life is.

I'M HEALED!!! You can be healed, too. No one has to be sick!

Epilogue

When I learned that natural healing offered so many answers to so many illnesses and diseases, I was so very excited. But a part of me was very angry because I saw the medical profession causing so much unnecessary suffering, refusing to use alternative methods that worked where their treatments failed. I was so angry, I even let it take me over at times.

Since working with patients, I have seen what this anger can do to people. One of my natural teachers would proclaim loudly, "Forgive the doctors!" and then in the next sentence, would declare how godless and evil medicine was. It was not my intention to write this story so that people can see how godless and evil medicine is. It is not my place to judge. Yes, I have seen better methods of healing disease than what the traditional medical establishment has to offer. But, at the same time, I do not believe that we as a country can entirely eliminate this form of medicine. It is not without its merits.

There are times when people really and truly need to see a medical doctor - sometimes for trauma (medical doctors are very good in this area of medicine), and sometimes, patients won't believe in anyone else because of their upbringing. Lastly, some people need to depend on the medical system to fix them as much as possible when they decide to drink excessively and smoke and otherwise slowly commit suicide by following such a horrible lifestyle that they cannot help but to suffer horrible diseases and eventually die from them. Natural healing has no "cures" for people who do not choose to be well.

In my healing work, I have noticed two types of people. There were those that just wanted to get on with healing. They asked questions about the healing routines and filled up their time thinking about it. They wanted to know what else they could do - what other books could they read? What other routines could they do? They were the ones who got their healing.

Then, there were the ones who wanted to tell me all day long how their doctor had wronged them or was still wronging them. They wanted to talk about medical conspiracies and about purposeful wrong acts. Since totally stopping the medical intervention all at once would have been dangerous, they struggled with continuing to go to a doctor that they considered to be incompetent and malicious. They believed this when it was the doctors who were in charge of the very therapies that were saving their lives. Their anger destroyed the relationship they had with their doctors and caused so much stress and anxiety, it caused their diseases to worsen. They were actually sabotaging their recovery.

I had inadvertently contributed to the second type of patient with my own anger at the medical establishment. Although I had many wonderful friends who taught me so much about natural healing, I had also surrounded myself with people who were **plenty** angry at the medical profession. I saw it wreak havoc on my life, as well as on the lives of patients. They were merely a reflection of my own anger. I eventually saw these angry people as having ideals incongruent with my own, and realized that if I wanted to teach people about natural healing, I would have to teach about love and forgiveness most of all.

As I worked on loving and forgiving all those in my life, those hateful, angry people just fell away. I was no longer able to relate to them or to their anger and did not wish to continue associating with them. What we think about and talk about all day may shape our entire experience of life. We may even **become** what we talk about and think about all day. I've made a new choice - I no longer choose to live my life in the negative. I don't want to talk about conspiracies. I want to talk about love.

I have seen plenty of natural healers who got into natural healing because natural healing saved their life. But they couldn't heal up all the way because they couldn't let go of their anger against the medical profession for "What they did to me." What the doctors "Did to them" was compel them to go into natural healing, and hopefully force them to have a better life because of it. What is wrong with that?

Everyone is a blessing to us in some way or another if we will only take the time and the courage to figure it out. There is nothing wrong with anger. It is a very valid emotion. To feel it is quite normal and understandable in such circumstances. And it should be expressed, because repressed anger also causes diseases. But once it's expressed, we cannot hold onto it forever - we have to let it pass like all of the other emotions we have from day to day. Ten and twenty year old grudges are very hard on the body.

I do not wish for people to go about using my story as ammunition against their doctors. I always feel that the relationship between doctor and patient is very important - if you feel your doctor is incompetent, either find a different way to look at it - maybe he is not so incompetent after all - he's been keeping you alive this long. Or, find a doctor that you **can** believe in. Don't just stay in the middle of the conflict and continue to let your anger eat you up. This is counter to the principles of natural healing. Natural healing is about being at peace with the situation at hand - with any and all situations - not just the ones that go the way you want them to go.

I do not wish for the medical establishment and the natural healers to be enemies. We are all cut from the same cloth. Don't all of us want to help? I wouldn't have written the story if I did not believe in the possibility of the medical profession to heal itself of its problems. I believe that medical doctors want to help. I believe in the possibility that we can all work together to make it happen somehow. I believe there will be a day for medicine that, conventional or otherwise, is kind, helpful, caring, empowering, inspiring, and healing. I live for that day.

Books etc.

Dangers of Medicine

1.   Confessions of a Medical Heretic, Robert S. Mendelsohn, M.D. Contemporary Books, Inc. An expose of the medical industry written by a prominent medical doctor (now deceased) who served on the Illinois Medical Licensure Committee, held many faculty and hospital posts and was the former director of Chicago's Michael Reese Hospital. It will open your eyes as to what is going on in the medical industry today. He states that if 95% of the medical industry disappeared, the health of the entire country would improve dramatically. He advocates as little medical care as possible by medical doctors.

2.   Dangers of Compulsory Immunizations, Family Fitness Press, Box 1658, New Port Richey, Florida 33552. How to legally avoid them.

3.   Vaccines: Are They Safe & Effective?, Neil Z. Miller. New Atlantean Press, P.O. Box 9638, Santa Fe, NM 87504.

4.   Immunizations: The Terrible Risks You Face That Your Doctor Won't Reveal. Robert S. Mendelsohn, M.D., Second Opinion Publishing, 1993.

5.   How To Raise A Healthy Child... In Spite Of Your Doctor, Robert Mendelsohn, MD, Ballantine Books, New York. Including chapters such as "How doctors can make healthy kids sick", and what to do when your child has an accident, cut, sprain, poisoning, etc.

6.   The Ultimate Rape: What Every Woman Should Know About Hysterectomies and Ovarian Removal, Elizabeth Plourde, M.T., M.A., New Voice Publications, P.O. Box 14133, Irvine, CA 92623.4133. Why NOT to have any of your female organs removed. Some of the results of having a hysterectomy: high blood pressure, atherosclerosis,

bowel and bladder problems, weight gain, depression, death, loss of sexual enjoyment, fibromyalgia, and osteoporosis, and more. Written by a medical technologist and very well researched.

Dangers Of Animal Products:

1.   Diet For A New America, John Robbins. Stillpoint Publishing. John Robbins, heir to the Baskin Robbins ice cream empire, leaves the industry and instead goes into research on the state of the animal raising industry. He describes in detail how the animals are raised, fed, and treated in horrible, shocking and unsanitary ways. He puts forth research supporting the benefits of a vegan diet and also addresses the issue of adequate protein, calcium and iron in a vegan diet in a very scientific manner supported by research. This book will make you never want to go near meat again (or any other animal product).

2.   Mad Cowboy: Plain Truth From The Cattle Rancher Who Won't Eat Meat, Howard F. Lyman, Scribner, New York. A former cattle rancher and feedlot operator, now considered the country's expert on mad cow disease, tells his story of how he and other feedlot operators raised foods and animals by using unnatural methods such as hormones, antibiotics, pesticides, etc, many of which had been banned. It will make you never want to eat   animal products again. Well researched.

3.   Don't Drink Your Milk! New Frightening Facts About The World's Most Overrated Nutrient, Frank A. Oski, M.D., TEACH Services, Inc., Brushton, New York, 1995.

Vegetarianism/Cookbooks

1.   The American Vegetarian Cookbook From The Fit-For-Life Kitchen, Marilyn Diamond, Warner Books, 1990. Excellent, practical cookbook including great-tasting substi-

tutions for animal products. Excellent book for those just making the transition to a vegetarian diet including a glossary of terms for health foods and how to stock a vegetarian pantry.

2.   May All Be Fed, John Robbins, William Morrow and Company, Inc., 1992. Very good vegan cookbook.

3.   The Uncheese Cookbook, Joanne Stepaniak, Book Publishing Company, Summertown, Tennessee, 1994. For those wishing to create cheesy-tasting dishes without the cheese. All dairy-free recipes.

4.   The New McDougall Cookbook, John A McDougall, MD, the Penguin Group, New York, New York.

5.   Vegan Nutrition: Pure & Simple, Michael Klaper, MD, Gentle World, Inc., PO Box 110, Paia, Maui, Hawaii 96779.

6.   Cookbook For People Who Love Animals, Gentle World, Inc., PO Box U, Paia, Maui, Hawaii 96779. Vegan cookbook. Contains no sugar or honey.

7.   Not Milk... Nut milks!, Candia Lea Cole. What to feed your child and yourself instead of milk. Over 50 recipes including almond milks, pecan milks, walnut milks, pine nut milks, sesame seed milks, pumpkinseed milks, sunflower seed milks, and cashew milks. YUM!

8.   Vegetarian Cooking School Cookbook, Danny and Charise Vierra, TEACH Services, Inc., Brushton, New York. Vegan recipes, the theories behind why to eat vegetarian, the dangers of animal foods (in detail), dangers of processed foods. Very well researched.

9.   Food For Life, Neal Barnard, M.D., Three Rivers Press, New York. Vegan cookbook.

10.   Dean Ornish's Program For Reversing Heart Disease, Ballantine Books, New York 1991.

Raw and Living Foods/Cookbooks
1.   *The Hippocrates Diet and Health Program, Ann Wig-

more. Avery Publishing Group, Inc. Raw food recipes as well as explanations of why a raw food diet and wheatgrass are so healing.

2. The Sprouting Book, Ann Wigmore, Avery Publishing Group, Inc., Wayne, New Jersey. The benefits of raw food and sprouts and how to easily make sprouts at home.

3. The Wheatgrass Book, Ann Wigmore, Avery Publishing Group, Garden City Park, New York. Detailed information on the benefits of wheatgrass and its juice, and how to grow wheatgrass at home.
   Living Foods For Optimum Health, Brian Clement with Theresa Foy Digeronimo, Prima Publishing, Rocklin, California, 1998.

4. Warming Up To Living Foods, Elysa Markowitz, Book Publishing Company, Summertown, Tennessee, 1998.

Juicing Books

1. The Complete Book of Juicing, Michael T. Murray, N.D. Prima Publishing. Contains many great-tasting juice combinations. Takes all the guesswork out of "What fruits and vegetables do I juice? The best, most practical juicing book I've seen.

2. Juicing for Life, Cherie Calbom, Maureen Keane. Avery Publishing Group, Inc. A good juicing book.

3. Juicing Therapy, Bernard Jensen, Bernard Jensen Enterprises.

4. Fresh Vegetable And Fruit Juices, N.W. Walker, D. Sc., Norwalk Press, Prescott, Arizona, 1978.

5. The Juiceman's Power Of Juicing, Jay Kordich (the "Juiceman"), William Morrow and Company, Inc., New York, 1992. Also, any other books he has written.

Emotional Healing

1. You Can Heal Your Life, Louise Hay, Hay House, Inc.,

Carson, California. Healing your life through your beliefs, emotions, and affirmations. Includes a section on the particular emotions and beliefs that are associated with and contribute to specific health problems.

2. Manifesto For A New Medicine, James S. Gordon, MD., Addison-Wesley Publishing Company, Inc., 1996. Mind-Body Medicine.
3. Ageless Body, Timeless Mind, Deepak Chopra, M.D., Three Rivers Press, New York, 1993.
4. Love, Medicine, and Miracles, Bernie S. Siegel, MD, HarperPerennial, New York, NY 1998.

Herbal and Natural Healing Books

1. Herbal Renaissance, by Stephen Foster. How to grow your own herbs.
2. Nontoxic, Natural, & Earthwise, Debra Lynn Dadd, Jeremy P. Tarcher, Inc. How to avoid toxic chemicals in our households (cleaners, deodorizers, polishes, insecticides, etc.) What easy natural alternatives to use instead, from natural products in the health food store to homemade solutions.
3. The Nontoxic Home and Office, Debra Lynn Dadd. Jeremy P. Tarcher, Inc. The sequel to #2.
4. Doctor-Patient Handbook, Bernard Jensen, D.C. Bernard Jensen Enterprises. The basics of healing and "healing crises". What to expect during a "cleanse".
5. Tissue Cleansing Through Bowel Management, Bernard Jensen, D.C. and Sylvia Bell, Bernard Jensen Enterprises. Shows the link between the condition of your bowels and your overall health. Great pictures showing all of the hardened accumulated waste that was drawn out of the bowels during cleansing procedures and pictures of people with diseases before and after the bowel cleansing. The results are dramatic.
6. Why Christians Get Sick, Rev. George H. Malkmus.

Destiny Image Publishers, Inc.

7. <u>School of Natural Healing</u>, Dr. John R. Christopher, Christopher Publications, Springville, UT. Excellent large reference book of herbal formulae, remedies, diseases, natural healing routines.

8. <u>The New Holistic Herbal</u>, David Hoffman, Element Books, Inc. Herbs for the different systems of the body: the circulatory, respiratory, digestive, nervous, skin muscular and skeletal, glandular, reproductive, urinary, and herbs for infections, cancer, the eyes, ears, nose and throat. A good section on how to make herbal preparations at home.

9. <u>The Scientific Validation of Herbal Medicine</u>, Daniel B. Mowry, Ph.D., Keats Publishing, Inc. For those scientifically- minded individuals who need proof and research of the effectiveness of herbs.

10. <u>Medicinal Plants</u>, (part of the Peterson Field Guide Series), Steven Foster/ James A. Duke, Houghton Mifflin Company. A field guide to identifying therapeutic plants/herbs.

11. <u>Your Body's Many Cries For Water</u>, F. Batmanghelidj, M.D., Global Health Solutions, Inc., Falls Church, VA 1997. Tells how many common ailments are due to dehydration.

12. <u>Rolfing - Stories of Personal Empowerment</u>, Briah Anson, North Atlantic Books, Berkeley, California, 1998.

13. <u>Bragg Healthy Lifestyle</u>, Paul C. Bragg, N.D., Ph.D., and Patricia Bragg, N.D., Ph.D., Health Science, Santa Barbara, California.

14. <u>Cancer Salves: A Botanical Approach To Treatment</u>, Ingrid Naiman, North Atlantic Books

15. <u>The Grape Cure</u>, Johanna Brandt, Benedict Lust Publications, New York, 1971.

16. <u>How I Conquered Cancer Naturally</u>, Eydie Mae with Chris Loeffler, Avery Publishing Group, Garden City

Park, New York, 1992.
17. Spontaneous Healing, How To Discover Your Body's
Natural Ability to Maintain and Heal Itself, Andrew
Weil, M.D., Ballantine Books,

Videos

1.   Question of Faith -a movie now in video stores. It is
about a woman (played by Ann Archer) diagnosed with lymphoma (cancer of the lymph nodes), who searches for alternative methods of healing. Excellent.

Iridology

1.   The Science and Practice of Iridology, Bernard Jensen, Bernard Jensen Enterprises, California.
2.   Iridology: The Science and Practice in the Healing
Arts, Bernard Jensen, Bernard Jensen Enterprises, California. Top of the line iridology text with many full color pictures of irises and explanations of the iris markings. Bernard Jensen is considered one of the fathers of iridology.
Excellent for practitioners as well as anyone else willing to
learn.

Anatomy

1   Atlas of the Human Body, Takeo Takahashi, Harper
Perennial. Excellent, clear,   anatomy pictures for those
lay persons interested in learning about their own anatomy
in order to empower themselves. Good explanations of each
system of the body. Best anatomy book for the lay person
that I've found.

Retreats/ Spas

1.   Hippocrates Health Institute – 1443 Palmdale Court,
West Palm Beach, FL 33411. Telephone: 561-471-8876.
Reservations only: 800-842-2125. Fax: 561-471-9464.

Web site: http://www.hippocratesinst.com.
2.   Optimum Health Institute of San Diego - 6970
Central Ave. Lemon Grove, CA 91945-2198. Telephone: 619-464-3346. Fax: 619-589-4098. Web site:
www.optimumhealth.org.
3.   Optimum Health Institue of Austing – R.R. 1 Box
3391, Cedar Creek, TX 78612. Telphone (512) 303-4817
or (512) 332-0106. Flgj73a@prodigy.com.
4.   Yoga Oasis - P.O. Box 1935, Pahoa, HI 96778.
Telephone: 800-274-4446 or 808-936-3727.Web site:
www.yogaoasis.org

Organic Food By Mail
1.   Gold Mine Natural Food Co. - 3419 Hancock St.,
San Diego, CA 92110-4307
2.   Diamond Organics - P.O. Box2159, Freedom, CA
95019. 1-888-ORGANIC (674-2642). Web page: http://
www.diamondorganics.com. For FRESH organic fruits
and vegetables - even wheatgrass, sprouts and edible
flowers. Also, organic pastas, breads, nuts, and dried
fruits.

PUBLISHER'S NOTE

Break On Through Press, LLC looks forward to publishing Dr. Foster's next two books over the coming 24 months.

The next book will be a comprehensive, yet simplified health program for those seeking specific methods of natural healing. It will include information on foods that harm and foods that heal, disease vs. detoxification (how to systematically clean each organ), tuning into your inner voice, methods of emotional and spiritual healing, how to determine your herbal doses, balancing the immune system, changing your body's chemistry through foods, juicing, herbs and hydrotherapy, the early warning signs of toxicity, how to stock your own herbal cabinet, and much, much more!

The third book in this series will be a splendid cookbook, with wonderful recipes to be used during herbal detoxification, as well as great-tasting recipes to build and maintain health every day!

We at Break On Through Press, LLC are always available for any questions or comments you have regarding any of our publications.

_P l e a s e   c o n t a c t   u s   a t :_

Contact Dr. Cynthia Foster at
PO Box 34693
Los Angeles, CA 90034-0693
drcfoster@earthlink.net
www.DrFostersEssentials.com